THE
TENTH
D◉OR

Dear Carol,

" Toward the One "

Peace Harmony, well-being,

Michele Hébert

THE
TENTH

D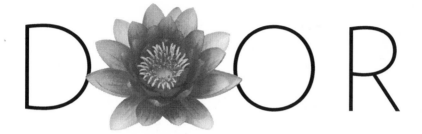OR

A Yoga Adventure

MICHELE HÉBERT

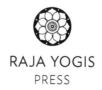

RAJA YOGIS

PRESS

Published by Raja Yogis Press
La Jolla, CA
www.RajaYogis.net

Distributed by Raja Yogis Press. 858-459-0880.

Design and composition by Greenleaf Book Group and Judythe Sieck
Cover design by Greenleaf Book Group

Publisher's Cataloging-In-Publication Data
(Prepared by The Donohue Group, Inc.)
Hébert, Michele.
   The tenth door : a yoga adventure / Michele Hébert.—1st ed.
   p. ; cm.
   ISBN: 978-0-9970366-0-2
   1. Hebert, Michele—Religion. 2. Spiritual life—Buddhism. 3. Hatha yoga.
4. El Salvador—History—20th century. I. Title.
BQ5670 .H43 2011
294.3444   2010934922

Printed in the United States of America on acid-free paper

15 16 17 18 19 20   10 9 8 7 6 5 4 3 2 1

Third Edition

For my teachers Walt and Magaña Baptiste
and
For Lisa, Marty, Kate, and Max

CONTENTS

The Tenth Door: There are nine physical openings in the
body. But there is a secret spiritual opening at the
crown of the head known as the tenth door.
It is from here that the spiritual adept
is trained to consciously leave
the body.

INTRODUCTION

This book is the story of my spiritual training with Raja Yoga Master Walt Baptiste, much of which took place in solitude in the jungles of El Salvador as that country moved from seeming tranquility to full-on revolution.

It has taken me more than twenty years to put this story down on paper. Over the years, I would occasionally try to tell my family, my friends, or my students about the incredible things that happened, but my attempts fell far short of the full truth. I realized that during the time I was having these esoteric experiences—all of which seemed perfectly normal to me—most people my age were holding down traditional jobs, buying houses, getting married, and raising families. I feared they could no more relate to my reality than they could to the man on the moon.

Besides, Life, as it is wont to do, got in the way of writing. After stepping back into the "real" world, I became immersed in teaching yoga, meditation, and mind-body health, and because of the quality and depth of these practical spiritual teachings, paths opened up to me that took me and my attention to the far reaches of the globe.

As I look back now, I realize that another reason for this long incubation period was that it has taken me this long to fully digest the incredible life-changing practices and lessons given to me by my amazing teacher and spiritual guide.

There is a wonderful story about the Buddha on his death-bed. His devotees were around him, and one summoned the courage to ask him who he was.

"Are you God?" asked the disciple.

"No," replied the Buddha.

"Are you just a man?"

"No," answered the Buddha.

"Then who are you?"

"I am awake," answered the Buddha.

And so it is: spiritually realized men and women come to us to help us wake up to our true essential nature. It is my hope that my story of awakening will inspire you on your own unique path of spiritual practice. We are, after all, one.

Michele Hébert
La Jolla, California

PART I

The Practical Mystic

CHAPTER 1

FULL MOON

El Salvador, 1977

"*Señorita Michele! Señorita Michele!*" The urgent whisper at my cabana window pulls me out of my slumber. Anna, the wife of our *guardián*, Fernando, is gesturing for me to follow her. The light of the full moon pours through the window screen. The full moon! I had noticed it earlier in the evening. Noticed, but not paid attention. I had merely brushed the thought away as if it were only a mosquito. I told myself that this time everything would be fine.

For three months I've been here in the remote jungles of El Salvador, on a few acres of beach property bordered by the Pacific. I've taken on the job of property manager at a spiritual retreat being built by Walt Baptiste, my teacher, and have been given the responsibility of readying the grounds and the buildings of *Retiro Espiritual* for groups of students who will come from the Baptiste Yoga Center in San Francisco. Most of my days have passed uneventfully. I've been alone except for the company of Anna the housekeeper, her husband and retreat caretaker Fernando, their two young daughters, and the construction workers who come during the day. Aside from performing my duties, I've had a great deal of time for meditation and other yoga practices. Most nights have been peaceful, too. Except for those with full moons.

My short experience with Fernando and full moons hasn't been good. The first full moon after Walt left me in charge, Fernando rode his bicycle around in circles for hours, laughing hysterically like the proverbial lunatic. His antics had awakened me after midnight, and when I tried to get him to stop he looked past me with a glassy expression that let me know he didn't register my presence. Twenty-eight nights later, he and a group of native men gathered around a large bonfire drinking Tic Tac, a cheap rotgut liquor, cavorting around the flames as if carrying out a ritual sacrifice. I have tried to tell myself it was coincidence, that there was no full moon mania pattern. Now, it seems that this night is already proving me wrong.

Outside my window, Anna is gesturing wildly. Moving quickly, I throw on shorts and a T-shirt, open the door, and step out into the sultry night. The roar of the ocean is deafening and I strain to hear her words.

"What is it, Anna? *Qué pasa?*" I ask, and then listen attentively as she carefully chooses the Spanish words she hopes I will understand.

"Fernando is very drunk. *Tiene un rifle.*" I manage to register enough words to slowly grasp the severity of the situation. *Neighbor's casita. Something about a rifle. Señor Baptiste's rifle.* I think she's trying to tell me that Fernando is in some kind of a fight. Anna frantically points in the direction of a hut on the property bordering ours. I know the owners of that property are gone for the season, but they keep employees—including their own caretaker—on the premises. To make matters worse, Raul Ortega, their caretaker, is feared by all of the local natives for his reputation of violence; he once chopped off a man's arm in a drunken machete fight. All the men carry machetes down here, the way Americans carry ballpoint pens.

Oh dear God, I think. *What should I do?* My Spanish is laughable. I've had minimal interaction with the natives, and I've never held a gun in my life. And yet, I've been given the responsibility of managing the retreat property, and my charge includes the safety of my surroundings and the people in it.

Fear and self-doubt set my mind spinning. All I can think of is a list of terrifying scenarios. But suddenly, Walt's voice comes into my head so strongly and clearly that I could have been talking on the phone with him. "Michele, calm down, go over there, and get that gun." I quickly look around to see if perhaps, by some extraordinary circumstance, my guru had returned from San Francisco to surprise me, but no, I am still alone. His physical body is nowhere in sight, but his presence—and most of all, his voice—is clearly with me.

I'm scared, I think.

Walt's reply comes immediately. "You will be protected."

Then, seemingly out of nowhere, my well-practiced mantra comes into my mind and repeats itself. *Peace, harmony, well-being. Peace, harmony, well-being.* As I experience the familiar words of the Baptiste teachings, I begin to calm down and feel my breath. I listen carefully for more inner guidance that might come. *Peace, harmony, well-being.* "You must control your own mind or negativity will." How often I heard my teacher say this in yoga class as he taught us to take responsibility for our states of mind. "When the mind calms," Walt said, "higher thinking is reflected, and the light from above is reflected." *Peace, harmony, well-being.*

I immediately feel a profound inner shift. The shadow of fear dissolves into the light of certainty. With absolute conviction, I stride to the neighboring property and open the collapsing wooden gate leading toward the dilapidated hut. None of the women in the neighbor's household are in sight, and Anna has not accompanied me. In this remote location, it is not uncommon to see men with missing hands or limbs lost in a machete fight. The women know all too well to stay away when things take an ugly turn.

I move toward the open door of the hut. Inside, I can see a bare mattress, a crude wooden table, a lantern, and two chairs. Several empty bottles of Tic Tac lie in a corner on the hard dirt floor. I can hear three men laughing wildly, but it's the kind of laughter that tells you nothing is funny. Then the laughter stops abruptly. Raul Ortega, the inhabitant of the hut, is attempting to stay on his feet as he slices his machete through the air like a sword. It slips from his hands and flies through the air, landing only inches from Fernando. Now, with both hands, Raul picks up a wooden chair and lifts it overhead, sending it careening into the chest of the man I do not recognize. The stricken man stumbles, grazing his shoulder on the small wooden table as he falls. The bare light of the kerosene lantern allows me to identify Fernando, pointing a rifle at Raul. I see well enough to note the menace in Fernando's eyes. This is no macho pose or drunken boast; this is real.

Taking a deep breath, I step through the door into air thick with kerosene and cheap alcohol.

"*Buenas noches,*" I say solemnly. The three men regard me

with complete and utter shock. I'm a girl, a *gringa*, in shorts no less. *"Hola, Señorita Michele,"* Fernando finally replies, lowering the rifle with a semi-remorseful look—not for his action, but for getting caught. The *guardián* of the adjoining property follows suit, attempting to show a measure of respect despite his drunkenness. Fortunately, he's coherent enough to recognize me as Walt Baptiste's representative, the retreat manager. Both his son and nephew had worked on the retreat, and jobs are scarce in this remote area.

The man on the floor is only semiconscious. I stand as tall as I can, with all the calm authority that my twenty-eight years can muster. Inwardly, my heart is hammering and I pray for strength. I have to be very careful. I don't want to shame Fernando in front of the other two men, and yet I know I have to get that gun.

"Please, Fernando, give me the gun. It belongs to Señor Baptiste."

"Señor Baptiste gave me this gun. I am the *guardián*," he protests, unable to meet my gaze.

"Only to defend the retreat property." I fumble with my limited Spanish vocabulary for the words that will convey to him the severity of the situation. I remain steadfast in my determination to get that gun.

Fernando stares at me sheepishly through an alcoholic haze. His guilty expression speaks volumes. He clearly knows, even in his inebriated condition, that he has broken a great trust. Looking down at the ground, he reluctantly hands me the weapon. I grasp it in both hands. Raul, looking relieved, flops backward onto his mattress, overcome by drink. I quickly walk out the door without looking back.

For the remainder of the night I lie in bed wide-eyed, with

Walt Baptiste's rifle under my bed. But I know that the gun is not what shields me from danger. *Peace, harmony, well-being. Peace, harmony, well-being.* Over and over I silently repeat the mantra that I had been given by Walt to defend my mind against fear and to help me abide in the knowingness that I am divinely protected. In the early morning hours I finally drift off to sleep as the words continue to slowly echo in my mind and into my dream state: *Peace, harmony, well-being.*

CHAPTER 2

OUT OF THE SNOW

"We must be willing to get rid of the life we've planned, so as to have the life that is waiting for us."
—JOSEPH CAMPBELL

*I*f anyone had told me when I was coming of age in Cleveland in the 1950s and 60s that I would spend four years of rigorous spiritual training with a yoga master in the jungles of El Salvador, I would have thought they were crazy. No one would have been more shocked than my elementary school teachers, the sisters of the Order of St. Ursula. My earliest religious training gave me little satisfaction or insight, although I was very good at memorization, learned the Catechism, and had a vague idea of the concept of divine omnipresence.

"Who made you?"

"God made me."

"Who is God?"

"God," I would dutifully reply, "is the creator of all things."

Yet, as early as I can recall, I felt that there was more to the whole idea of divine presence than I was being taught in school. In a secret place inside I knew it, I felt it, and I longed for it. My parents dutifully passed on their Roman Catholic heritage to me even before my schooling began, and by the age of two

I believed with conviction that I was a child of God with a guardian angel who was always by my side. Wherever I went, my guardian angel went, too. I pictured my angel as the number-one angel of them all: Michael, the archangel.

At night, when my mother or father tucked me into bed, we said a special prayer.

> *Angel of God, my guardian dear,*
> *To whom God's love commits me here;*
> *Ever this day be at my side,*
> *To light and guard, to rule and guide. Amen.*

My parents also told me that when people died, they went to God and lived in heaven with the angels. This comforted me. Life was safe and good. I was surrounded by my parents, by angels, and by God, all of whom would protect me from harm.

One cold and snow-blown Cleveland day when I was four, I had a chance to test my fledgling sense of faith. My mother bundled my younger brother Britt and me in snowsuits, scarves, hats, and boots, and sent us out to the backyard to play. In the aftermath of a giant blizzard, the mounds of snow created from my father's shoveling were over five feet high. I intrepidly scaled one cold, white mountain while my brother wandered over to another part of the yard. Suddenly, my foot slipped and I fell headfirst into the snow pile. Only my red boots stuck out from the cave my body had created. I frantically called out for my brother and waited expectantly, hoping he had seen my mishap. It was cold, wet, and dark inside the snowdrift, and as the minutes slowly passed, it occurred to me that perhaps no one would find me. Perhaps I would die here.

Curiously, I wasn't at all frightened. I accepted my fate calmly.

I was beginning to get sleepy, though, and mused dreamily of floating among the angels in heaven. Death would gently take me to a bright and beautiful place. Maybe I would even become an angel.

But this was not my time to go. I was pulled out of my white reverie by a tugging sensation on one of my legs. I heard a muffled, childlike voice. Britt had recognized my boots, understood my situation, and was digging me out, pulling my legs as hard as he could to deliver me back to the world. I hugged him and thanked him for saving me, delighted to have the chance to continue my life. I was now more secure than ever in the understanding that dying was not to be feared. At the same time, the episode of falling into a giant snowbank was not one I wanted to repeat. I ran breathlessly into the kitchen to tell my mother about my close call. She wrapped her arms around me as I buried my head in the warm safety of her soft breast.

At St. Ann's Elementary School, where the subject of religion was given a prime morning slot, none of my spiritual inklings catapulted me to the head of the class. As a student, I was something of a scatterbrain. I spent a lot of time doodling—mostly pictures of triangles and a strange and exotic flower whose name and significance I would not find out for many years. I also managed to regularly irritate the presiding sister by consistently forgetting my black doily chapel veil on the twice-weekly Mass days. A paper napkin was substituted and tacked onto my head with a bobby pin so the entire world could bear witness to my absentmindedness. Mass itself became—as you can imagine—something of a fashion nightmare, but it was also a mental torment. Having to sit quietly and listen to the priest speaking Latin for a half hour gave my mind little to latch onto. Each Mass seemed like an eternity as I struggled between daydreaming and pretending to be attentive and pious. It wasn't until I began the rosary contest with my friend Betsy Johnson that I found a personal purpose amidst the rituals.

My goal in each Mass became getting through as many rosaries as possible and trying to outdo Betsy. It was the perfect game because no one else could possibly imagine what was going on. It didn't require the two of us even looking at one another. I amazed myself with how fast I could tear through those rosary prayers. The trick was to not hesitate even for a second between prayers, so that all sixty prayers ran together like one long incantation. On a good day, I could get through more than four rosaries in thirty minutes. Betsy and I were often neck and neck, although I basked in the glory of holding a slight lead at the end of the school year. In a way, I now believe, I was already training for the ancient yogic practice of using *malas*, strings of prayer beads, to hone my attention. The *malas* worn and used by yogis and Buddhists for thousands of years consist of 108 beads. In the Yoga tradition, a mantra or sacred word is repeated silently as each bead is fingered. The practice is used to help control the mind and keep it focused in a positive and spiritual direction, ultimately serving as a tool to foster the continual awareness of God's presence. The Catholic rosary practice is based on the same idea. But all I knew at the time was that it helped me fend off third grade restlessness.

Sometimes, in class and in Mass when my attention appeared to be wandering, I think the people around me would have been surprised to know where it had wandered. On many occasions, I was privately thinking about Jesus and his disciples and sometimes trying to imagine what it would be like to be one of Jesus's close followers. In fact, in moments of fervor, I was actually overtaken with remorse that I had been born too late to be a disciple.

But the Law of Karma, which can also be called the Law of Cause and Effect, will nudge even us scatterbrains toward our destiny. And its corollary, the Law of Reincarnation, also plays a role. The Law of Reincarnation, so called because it refers to reaping karma across multiple lifetimes, posits that even the family situations that we are born into are the result of past-life actions and of ties and relationships that need to be worked out in this lifetime. Looking back, I see that, in a way, I did spend part of my childhood as a disciple. I was, like my siblings, a disciple of my father—and our discipline was music.

My father, William Hébert, played flute and piccolo with the world-renowned Cleveland Orchestra for forty-one years and was considered one of the world's most accomplished flutists. As a child growing up in Boston, he had been stricken with tuberculosis and his mother, a nurse, had bought him a flute to strengthen his lungs. His family, victims of the Great Depression, was so poor and so large that scraping up the fee for a weekly lesson was an enormous challenge, and my father would have to hang off the back of a bus to get to his teacher's house because paying bus fare on top of it all was unthinkable. Yet he took to the flute with a passion that would never fade. He played in the U.S. Army band in the South Pacific, studied at Juilliard on a scholarship, and summoned every ounce of his courage, determination, and skill to successfully audition for Cleveland conductor George Szell. He also passed his love of music on to his own children.

At our house, it was simply a given that my five younger brothers and I would each study an instrument. We would often all be practicing at once, on three different floors of our house, making for quite the cacophony (my mother explicitly forbade the study of drums to keep her last nerve from shattering). I took flute lessons from my father for years, and with me, as with all his students, he set the highest of standards. But in addition to being my musical mentor, my father also guided me through innumerable lessons I would not come to fully appreciate, or fully apply, until much later. He taught me about the rewards of rigorous effort, and he taught me to strive for perfection. He also taught me how to breathe.

At the age of seven I asked my father if I could one day play the flute. The sound was a language of deep feeling and a sensuality that played on my heartstrings until the notes became a very part of me.

"When you are nine years old," he promised, "I will teach you to play the flute."

True to his word, on my ninth birthday I received a beautiful, shiny new instrument.

My first flute lesson was not at all what I had pictured. When you took your first flute lesson with William Hébert you did not, I discovered, under any circumstances play the flute. Instead, you lay on the floor while he put a hardcover *Webster's Unabridged Dictionary* on your solar plexus and instructed you in the proper way to inhale and exhale from your diaphragm. At first, I was restless to get to the flute, but when the heavy dictionary was placed on my diaphragm, it got my complete attention as I tried to use my breath to lift the weighty book and smoothly lower it with the exhalation.

"When can I take out the flute?" I pleaded.

"The flute is a wind instrument," he patiently explained. "Your breath is the wind and it is the foundation of playing. If your breath is weak, the sound will be weak. If the breath is strong and controlled, the sound you make on the flute will be strong. It's all about the breath. You must learn to breathe from your diaphragm first, and this exercise will train you to do that."

Little did I know that this first flute lesson was also my first lesson in yoga. Dad's emphasis on the breath and its energies and flow actually comprised my earliest teachings in *pranayama*, the ancient yogic science of controlling life energy via the breath to cleanse the body and clear the mind—a skill which would become of vital importance to me later in life.

But none of this occurred to me at the time, and as much as I enjoyed playing music I stopped my lessons with my father when I was sixteen. I'd discovered boys—not my brothers, but real boys—who can be very time consuming. I'd also discovered Marlboros—not so good for the breath at my rate of a pack a day. As a teenage girl who, for so long, had been the responsible big sister, I was ready to step out and party. In the great pantheon of iconic American teenage rebels, I wouldn't qualify as even a minor character, but for a Catholic schoolgirl from Cleveland, I indulged in my share of eyebrow-raising adventures when out of my parents' protective view.

By this time, all five brothers were on the scene, and my good-hearted mother was operating in "overwhelm" mode. Preparing three meals a day, driving someone or other to an after-school lesson, and trying to hold the fort down while my father was on tour for weeks on end were all herculean tasks. Needless to say, she yelled a lot. To make matters worse, she and I were constantly at odds. "You treat this house like a hotel," she would mutter, looking up over a meal she was preparing, as I waltzed through the kitchen and out the back door on my way to meet my friends, who understood me.

In the midst of such a busy household, I became a master at doing what I wanted while escaping detection. But there is a story still told in my family about "that New Year's Eve" when I failed, literally, to cover my tracks. I'd been escorted home by my boyfriend at my appointed curfew of 12:30 a.m. and politely greeted the guests at a party my parents were hosting before feigning fatigue and heading off to bed. Knowing that the guests' hubbub would cover any telltale creaking floorboards, I sneaked out the back door, met back up with my date, and went to a rowdy, all-night gathering of friends. When I returned home just before dawn, I found our house locked up tight and myself without a key. I thought I was clever when I found an unlatched door at a friend's house across the street and slept on the living room couch. But when I woke up at 9:00 a.m., snow had blanketed the neighborhood. How could I get back to my house without leaving footprints? Simple! I walked home backwards, and even when I noticed my father staring at me from my own third-floor bedroom window, I attempted to keep up my ruse by waving at an imaginary acquaintance and shouting, "Bye, bye. Nice to see you."

Needless to say, parents are never as witless as sixteen-year-olds imagine them to be (this, too, is a law of the universe), and mine were no exception. Although my antics continued, I started getting caught—a lot. I'd be caught with cigarettes. Grounded. Caught with a date when I was supposed to be studying. Grounded. Caught slipping out while being grounded. Double-grounded. The remainder of high school was a contest of wills that appeared to end with my parents getting me to agree to enroll in a Jesuit college, Marquette University in Milwaukee. I think they believed the Jesuits would save me, but the school had the opposite effect. I was an agnostic by my second week and never went to church. To make matters worse, when my beloved roommate announced she was getting engaged to her high school sweetheart and would be leaving school after the first semester of our sophomore year, out of pure insecurity

I decided to do the same. I moved back to Ohio to marry my high school love.

The marriage didn't last. How could it when it was based on my own immature motivation and the fact that everyone else seemed to be doing it? We were too young to know ourselves, much less understand the needs of the other. We stumbled through as best we could, but as soon as I finished college I left the marriage, emotionally devastated, and ran back to my Cleveland roots, where I slowly reassembled myself with the help of friends and family.

Despite my seemingly upbeat demeanor, a depression began to take hold of me that I could not shake. I used alcohol, male attention, and endless social engagements to deaden the nameless pain and began searching desperately for something outside of myself to give life some meaning. I found some decent jobs that earned me enough money to travel in Europe for a few aimless months, searching for I knew not what, but it was a lonely pilgrimage and I was relieved to return home, where at least I had a support system. Through friends I took a job as communications director with a candidate for Ohio lieutenant governor. I also applied to Case Western Reserve University for a master's degree in social work, although I secretly harbored some political ambitions of my own. I got a grant from Case Western and planned to attend. I badly wanted to reclaim some sense of identity, and becoming a student again gave me some semblance of direction. I almost believed how well things were falling into place. But in a large corner of my heart, I knew very well that this was my last effort to play the game of courting acceptance and approval, at which I had become adept in recent years.

One overcast Monday morning in 1974, the charade suddenly

ended. I awoke with a calm certainty that my life was headed in the wrong direction. I had no doubt, no confusion. There was no sense of running from anything, only a deep conviction that the next chapter of my life lay elsewhere. The grant I had won would have required me to work for the state of Ohio for five years after graduation. I knew that just wasn't going to happen. I felt an uncontrollable urge to leave Cleveland immediately.

This emotion was so powerful that I tried to brush it aside and go on to other thoughts. I had developed a delicious ritual of staying in my warm bed for a few minutes before getting up and allowing thoughts to simply flow through my mind. Sometimes they were thoughts related to recent events, and sometimes they were creative ideas. But this particular morning my mental musing session was not meant to be. I lay there paralyzed, a feeling of dread building until I was at its mercy. My inner sense of knowing shouted at me that I absolutely had to turn and run as fast as I could from a life that would be certain doom if I continued on my current path. Even so, I made a last attempt to stay the course.

"How can I walk away from my life here?"

Easy. Just do it, came the reply.

"Won't I be letting down my parents and all of the people who have supported me?"

They love you and want the best for you.

"How do I tell the university people that I am walking away from their generous grant?"

Tell them the truth.

"Where will I go, and what will I do?" There was a slight pause, and finally the answer came with joyous conviction.

CALIFORNIA!

California? Even I wondered if this wasn't a cliché. Had I been overexposed to the Beach Boys? Had I listened to that Mamas and Papas anthem once too often? *I'd be safe and warm if I was in L.A.* But then that voice came again and I knew. It could only be California. Clichés become truisms because they are so often true, I reminded myself. In mystical, ever-sunny California, *right at that moment* juicy oranges were being plucked from trees and coconut palms were swaying in the balmy breezes. Frothy ocean waves were crashing on white sandy beaches where beautiful tanned bodies frolicked by the sea. All the people there were infinitely cooler than I had so far ever had a prayer of being. And all those cool people were living the life of their dreams and having the time of their lives.

With my unusual wake-up call delivered, it was time for me to get practical. I tallied up the people I knew who lived in California: a friend in Santa Barbara, a cousin in Los Angeles, a high school friend in Sacramento. I added up the sum of money I could gather to launch me on my new life: four hundred dollars. How on earth was I going to *get* to California? The answer that popped up was truly a stroke of genius: the Cleveland Orchestra.

"Yes, that's it!" I exclaimed as I reached across the bed, picked up the phone, and promptly called my father. I knew his orchestra would be leaving the following week on a two-week tour of California. When he answered the phone, I broke the news to him, laying out my life-changing revelation. He listened quietly, as he always did, until I was finished. I ended with a simple request: "Can you get me on that plane?"

The moment of silence that followed seemed like an eternity. He knew me well. As the father of now seven children (my only sister was born when I was nineteen), he had spent twenty-six years guiding his eldest daughter and watching her move into adulthood and dive into life with reckless abandon.

He was always there as a safety net, fishing me out when I was in over my head. Despite our tussles, he became a bridge for me as I transitioned from my wildly independent teenage years through the missteps of my early adulthood. Although he often gave me advice and reeled me in when I strayed too far, he knew too well that I was determined and headstrong and tended to do what I wanted in the face of what I believed were unfair parental guidelines. Pressing the phone to my ear, I could practically hear my father weighing the possibilities and crafting a thoughtful response as I held my breath.

"I'll see what I can do," he replied.

And in that moment my fate was sealed. I let my breath go, and on some level swore I could feel my soul sigh with relief. Unbeknownst to me, at least on a conscious level, I was en route to meet my spiritual destiny—accompanied by 103 members of the esteemed Cleveland Orchestra.

CHAPTER 3

A TOE IN THE WATER

"Life is either a daring adventure or nothing."
—HELEN KELLER

*F*or me, the 1974 Cleveland Orchestra tour of California marked a pivotal transition, a time when my karma began rapidly unfolding. But it always makes me smile to remember that other people recall that tour as a cultural watershed of sorts.

During the orchestra's much-lauded appearance at the Hollywood Bowl, at just the moment when conductor Lorin Maazel raised his baton to begin the concert, a man ran across the stage. Except for a pair of socks, running shoes, and a paper bag over his head, this healthy young specimen was stark naked. On this night, the term "streaking" was introduced into America's vocabulary. *I'm a long way from Cleveland,* I thought.

The entire orchestral entourage stayed for one week at the luxurious Ambassador Hotel in Los Angeles. For me, it was like being at a large, festive family reunion, with the added joy of exposure to one high-level musical experience after another on a daily basis. I had grown up with these world-class musicians, and to me they were uncles and aunts. In fact, some of them had played at my Cleveland wedding six years earlier.

One day, at the hotel, I wandered into the fitness center and ended up taking my first yoga class. For years I had turned down my mother's repeated invitations to join her at her Jewish Community Center yoga classes. But suddenly, maybe because I was adopting the California spirit, I was eager to give it a try. I was amazed at how balanced and centered I felt after the class was over. Was this feeling I was experiencing what yoga was about? Could it be the purpose of yoga to help practitioners arrive at this wonderfully calm and clear state? I shook my head at my hundreds of stubborn refusals to participate.

As it happened, yoga was not the only thing to impact my state of mind on that particular day. In class, I'd struck up a conversation with two young men. Chatting with them around the pool later, I introduced them to my father and to my mother, who'd also come along on the tour. My new friends invited me to a party that night—a Hollywood party!—and I gladly accepted. At that party, while I was dancing, I started to feel very strange. My perceptions were heightened; all sensations were enhanced. I felt like I was literally "dancing my head off." Soon the secret was out: someone had spiked the punch with LSD. I know that I continued dancing (when in Rome . . .), but the rest of the party was a blur. When I got back to the hotel I used every ounce of will to appear perfectly normal while telling my parents that the party had been "very nice" and that I'd see them in the morning. Despite the prevalence of hallucinogenics in the 1970s, I'd never done anything like this. I was no angel, but I was more of a mixed drinks and Irish coffee kind of girl. But of my two mind-bending experiences that day, one thing was clear: I preferred the yoga.

A week later, I said tearful good-byes to my parents and spent two weeks visiting everyone I knew in California. I didn't have a clue where my final destination would be, but I felt sure that at some point on my journey I would know.

My first stop was to visit my cousin Jimmy, a UCLA law student living in Santa Monica. One glorious, quintessentially Californian afternoon, he took me on an outing.

"Where are we going?" I asked, as the car wound through an upscale residential neighborhood lined with perfectly symmetrical palm trees.

"Trust me, Michele," he replied. "You're going to love it. Just do me a favor. Leave your cigarettes in the car."

We ended up in spectacular Pacific Palisades at the Lake Shrine of the Self-Realization Fellowship. The Self-Realization Fellowship, I learned upon entering its gates, was a yoga organization that had many temples throughout the United States. This one was the jewel in its crown, a serene and enchanting spiritual sanctuary that was visited each year by thousands of people of all faiths. The now-deceased yoga master who founded the Fellowship, Paramahansa Yogananda, had introduced yoga to the West. It was reported that after he died, his body smelled like roses, and up to the time of his burial thirty days later, it never decomposed. The Lake Shrine grounds included a statuary garden. I stood, curious, before the statues and recognized one as Jesus. The other statues were of Yogananda and his lineage of teachers. As a renegade Catholic, I was mystified at Jesus's appearance here but I understood that he, too, was a renegade of sorts.

As Jimmy and I strolled around the lake, I was aware of becoming more and more relaxed, until I found myself in a blissful state of deep calm. The setting sun's reflection on the water created millions of twinkling diamond lights and I could almost see tiny water sprites dancing on them. We stopped and sat silently on a perfectly situated meditation bench facing the violet waters of the lake. When the time seemed right, we stood in unison and resumed our walk. It was as if all boundaries had melted away, leaving only serenity within and without. The past faded, all future thoughts stilled, and the movement of us walking together around this sparkling lake in the setting sun was all that existed.

When we circled the lake and arrived back at the statues, I stopped and silently studied them more closely. All of the faces exhibited great strength of character balanced with humility and kindness. They seemed to be communicating a hidden possibility that nothing in my previous experience would allow me to penetrate. As we turned to go back to the car, I made a mental note that when I finally settled down, I would look further into this yoga thing.

After a week at Jimmy's place, I went on to visit my old friend Rick, who was waiting tables in Santa Barbara. Rick and I had worked together on the last lieutenant governor's campaign in Ohio. When our candidate lost, he also decided to migrate west. Although Rick was working, I was not. And as beautiful as Santa Barbara was, I was bored. It only took me a few days to realize an aimless partying lifestyle was not for me, and I headed north to see a dear childhood friend, Marsha, in Sacramento.

Marsha had chosen a very different lifestyle than mine. In her early twenties, she had married the youngest judge in California and was the mother of a two-year-old girl. They lived in a large, beautiful home in the suburbs. During my stay in Sacramento, I accompanied Marsha on her weekly trip to San Francisco, where she was taking an art class. While she was in class, I jumped on a cable car and rode around and around the city marveling at the spectacular views and enjoying the friend-liness and free-spirit atmosphere that San Francisco exudes. I stumbled across a famous Irish coffee bar at Fisherman's Wharf and had fun chatting with a group of tourists from Michigan. I strolled through Chinatown and wandered through City Lights, a North Beach bookstore that was cofounded by the Beat poet Lawrence Ferlinghetti and was a favorite bohemian hangout. On my way back to meet Marsha, I hung off the bar of the cable car and let the wind whip through my hair as I reveled in a state of exhilaration. My decision was made. I knew I had found the place I wanted to be.

One problem: I was down to about two hundred dollars, and even in those days San Francisco had a relatively high cost of living, at least compared to Cleveland.

"Will you be okay?" Marsha asked as she dropped me off at my San Francisco hotel room the following week. "Call us if you need anything." She hugged me good-bye as I practically skipped to the door of the downtown residence club that I had chosen sight unseen. At that time, San Francisco was one of the few U.S. cities that even had residence clubs. They are similar to European pensions; rooms can be let weekly or monthly and include breakfast and dinner.

The Ansonia, just off Union Square, was filled to the brim with colorful characters. My roommate was a young African-American woman who informed me she was a witch—a good witch. *Hey,* I thought, *what the heck. It's San Francisco.* Another temporary resident turned out to work for the Mitchell broth-ers, cofounders of the O'Farrell Theatre, an "erotic emporium" that had become a major city attraction for residents and tour-ists alike. After staying at this pension for a week or two, I was running out of money, so I took a switchboard job there that

covered my room and board and paid twenty dollars for working fifteen hours a week. But it was clear I needed another
source of income.

Since I'd had some experience with political campaigns, I
answered a newspaper ad placed by a man who was running for
city supervisor. The man turned out to be Leonard Orr, who
had already achieved fame in another arena. He had made a
name for himself in the emerging human potential movement.
He was a teacher of metaphysics, well-known on the West
Coast for his "rebirthing" technique. I ended up getting the job,
in a way. Leonard felt that two other candidates and I each had
special qualifications, so he split the position three ways. One of
my two associates was a San Francisco deputy sheriff. The other
was a man who was about one year into an intensive two-year
therapy known for stripping its participants of all psychological
defenses before reconstructing them in what was supposed to
be a healthier way. At the halfway point, this devotee was filter-
free, unable or willing to edit anything that came out of his
mouth. Once again, like Dorothy in Oz, I had to remind myself,
"We're not in Cleveland anymore."

Not only was I on a great adventure, but now I could also
afford to sublet a small, furnished apartment on Sacramento
Street, a bit closer to the Golden Gate Park panhandle where
Leonard's Victorian mansion was located. My new neighborhood was charming, and I took to exploring it with long
morning walks. The first day, I passed by a man walking down
Arguello Boulevard dressed in all white, his head clean shaven,
his eyes sparkling. He smiled at me with so such warmth I felt
myself light up inside. It was an image that lingered long after
the moment ended. Was everyone around here so welcoming?

Working for Leonard turned out to involve a little bit of

everything. I worked on his campaign, but I also became acquainted with his rebirthing practice. Rebirthing techniques are still around today, and have come to be associated with specialized breathing techniques. But in Orr's pioneering method, you were immersed in a huge water tank (there was one in the basement of his Victorian house) and equipped with a snorkel. The original idea was that through a specific underwater breathing exercise, all sorts of latent emotional issues would surface so they could be resolved. I was actually rebirthed once, but I honestly don't remember much about the experience. Leonard came to trust me enough that he chose me to assist with his own rebirthing process. This involved standing in the tank with him as a supportive and grounding observer as he submerged himself in the tank for several minutes and breathed deeply through a snorkel.

Leonard was also a teacher of metaphysics and gave seminars on the power of the mind. The first time I accompanied him to one of these seminars, my mind was blown open. We flew to L.A., where the workshop was held at the beach home of one of his Santa Monica followers. He began by writing on a whiteboard the phrase "THOUGHT IS CREATIVE."

I immediately fluctuated between confusion and rebellion. *No way do my thoughts have anything to do with what happens in my life.* But the universe has its own way of teaching us its laws, and apparently Leonard was its vehicle to wake me up to Lesson One: Every thought we think is, in fact, creating our future.

Of all that Leonard exposed me to, I am also grateful for one other significant thing. He was a great proponent of deep breathing as a metaphysical tool. He himself was constantly breathing deeply and sighing loudly. One day he told me about a book that he said would help me greater understand the power of the breath. It was called *Autobiography of a Yogi* by Paramahansa Yogananda, the very yogi who had founded the Self-Realization Fellowship that I visited in L.A. with my cousin. In it, the great master teaches that it takes 150,000 lifetimes for a soul to reach enlightenment, and that we are given a certain number of breaths in each lifetime. When we use up our allotted number of breaths, our life ends. The accomplished yogi learns to conserve his breath—to breathe deeply and slowly rather than quickly and shallowly, thus living a long, full life. Reading this spiritual classic—part adventure story, part philosophical wisdom—affected me profoundly. And it served to remind me of the promise I'd made myself: look into the yoga thing.

Soon after, I found myself at a popular San Francisco restaurant, the Hungry Mouth, located on Clement Street, a few blocks from my new apartment. It was part of a large health complex that included a gym, dance studio, and yoga center. Wandering into the adjoining health food store, I noticed a posted ad for yoga instruction and had an inspiration.

Behind the counter was a slight Asian man wearing a white short-sleeved T-shirt that spelled out "Bee Power" in a circle on the front. He sported a Fu Manchu goatee and moved quickly, like a hummingbird. In front of him was a bag of miniature peanuts. "Chinese peanuts," he informed me, as he proceeded to shell one and pop it into his mouth with one hand as he handed me a carrot juice with the other. I took a deep breath and asked whether I could work at the Hungry Mouth in exchange for yoga classes.

"You'll have to talk to Walt," said the kind-eyed fellow behind the counter. "Why not go to tomorrow morning's yoga class and talk to him afterward?"

Okay, I thought gamely. *Why not? But who's this Walt?*

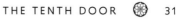

I downed the carrot juice in a few gulps and left with a spring in my step. I didn't know if the vitamin A had given me a boost or if something else was going on, but I felt on top of the world.

CHAPTER 4

WELCOME HOME

*T*he purpose of life," affirmed the teacher, "is to grow into the fullness and wholeness of all that we can be."

I cautiously opened one eye ever so slightly to peek at my surroundings. The gigantic carpeted yoga studio exuded an aura of royalty. Its ornately carved wood trim and red velvet couches, seemingly from another era, lined either side of the large meditation space. Cathedral-like opaque windows gave the room an ethereal light, and finely wrought exotic tapestries depicting scenes from Indian mythology hung in several places around the room. An elaborate stained-glass skylight with an ornate letter *G* at its center was embedded in the apex of a two-story ceiling.

I had chosen a yoga mat in the third row and viewed several attentive students in front of me, legs crossed, spines erect, and eyes closed. They appeared to be listening intently to the words of the yoga master, who sat facing us on a raised platform surrounded by flowers, gongs, flutes, and an array of richly colorful and ornate Eastern artifacts.

The teacher, a man in his fifties, had a shaven head, a large, muscular chest, and a powerful presence. His white slacks and freshly pressed white Nehru-style jacket added to his clear and peaceful affect. Sitting on a blue and white batik pillow, he seemed completely relaxed, despite the fact that his spine appeared unfalteringly straight. His ankles were crossed and his feet rested on a step below where he was seated. His small feet were encased in white cotton coverings that were more like mittens than socks.

His large, dark brown eyes were luminous and expressed great depth and wisdom.

It was obvious that he was at home with both the concepts he was teaching and his role as the teacher in this magnificent temple room. As he spoke, his arm gestures hypnotized me. They seemed to move in space with the speed of light but with the grace and precision of a trained dancer. He was effortlessly conscious of every part of himself.

My eye was only open for a few seconds when I saw Walt Baptiste looking directly into me. No, not *at* me, but rather, into the depths of me. Momentarily mesmerized, I looked into his eyes and met a clear and knowing gaze. Could it be . . . ? Was this the man who had dazzled me with his smile that day when I first moved into the neighborhood? I somehow knew it was. In that second, I realized that there was nowhere to hide from this man. He knew who I was. Self-conscious and overwhelmed, I quickly shut my eye, as if somehow this would protect me from being discovered. My brain raced through its files searching for a comparable experience, anything that would help me make sense of what was happening.

"In meditation," the teacher continued, "we close the two physical eyes and look inside with the eye of the mind." His tone was even and nonjudgmental, but I was certain he was directing his words specifically to me. As the discourse continued, I started to feel physically uncomfortable. My lower back began to ache in response to my unusual seated position. I temporarily forgot about my earlier anxiety as my focus of attention settled on my bodily woes. I contemplated a variety of ways in which I could remove myself from this scenario as quickly as possible. Did people here take bathroom breaks?

I thought about the large doorway behind me but realized that it would not be appropriate to just get up and walk out. It would make the statement that I was a quitter, and my ego would not permit that. But despite what I was going through, there was also an unknown force that compelled me to stay. The words of the teacher were inspirational, encouraging us to be the best that we could be within ourselves. And again, I could swear that he was talking directly to me.

Oh, well, I consoled myself. *It's only an hour of my life. It will be over soon.*

Time, however, had taken on a new dimension. It practically stood still. The minutes limped by and I began to wonder if this yoga and meditation class was going to go on forever. In fact, perhaps I would die in this position. My left leg was falling asleep and my straight spine had turned into a letter *C*. I could hardly concentrate on what was being said, I was in such a state of discomfort.

The teacher continued speaking in words that seemed to contain not only great wisdom but also a vast, unconditional love. But I had more immediate things to deal with—an aching body and a screaming mind. Since I'd ruled out total escape, in desperation I began plotting ways to quietly move my legs so that I would not be noticed.

"The person operating from a state of balance and wholeness

has a completely different life experience than the person coming out of weakness and imbalance."

No kidding, I thought. He was clearly speaking to me personally. But I no longer cared that I was being singled out. My left
leg was gone now. Where it went, I could not guess. How in
the world I would be able to stand up and walk out of the room
if the class ever ended I could not imagine. To an observer, it
might appear as if I was simply sitting quietly, but inside I was
on fire. I could not do it. My mind was in torment and my body
was rebelliously protesting, waving an internal placard reading,
Yoga class unfair! Must stop now! The crescendo was deafening. I
could not sit still another moment.

Somewhere in the distance, I could hear the teacher's voice
resonating calmly and compassionately. He seemed to know
exactly what I was experiencing and was intentionally guiding
me through my physical and mental anguish.

"Be the observer of the mind. Watch what you are doing
within yourself mentally and emotionally. You are not the mind;
you are something besides the mind. You are not the body; you
are something besides the body. You are pure consciousness.
You must learn not to be motivated out of pain, suffering, and
misery. Everything is inside you, from the lowest to the highest.
Choose wisely between the negative and positive poles of the
mind. Be of good counsel and repeat the words *peace, harmony,
well-being*, instead."

Peace, harmony, well-being. Peace, harmony, well-being. I clung to
these words and began repeating them over and over. At first
they were just words, but as I continuously repeated them, I
actually began to relax. The storm lifted. My tormented body
completely disappeared and I found myself in a state of pure
stillness, pure existence, without a second thought. My very

breath seemed to have stopped, although I was aware of a subtle inner energy flow that sustained me. I had entered a deep place inside myself and had no interest in relating to the antics of my mind or to the outer world. The peace within was far more compelling.

As I rested in this place, I became aware of what seemed like a field of moon glow encompassing my being. The teacher's far-off words guided me. "I want you to realize the divine light of your own soul within you. Your own inner light will reveal your soul's purpose. If you need further support, the guide will be there. I, as a spiritual guide, must not be shy about demanding what is required—I ask nothing of anyone in practice that I have not myself gone through. There must be this honesty or there is no spiritual master."

The class ended and the teacher left the room. I took a moment to massage my legs back to life and then followed to find him. Even though my legs had regained feeling I had the curious sensation that I was floating, not walking. I saw Walt standing under a nearby archway, talking to a small group of students.

He turned to me and I was vaguely aware that I was taller than he, which was surprising because he was so physically imposing. I was aware that there were other people within listening range, but I didn't care. Words began tumbling out of my mouth.

"Thank you," I said politely, holding out my hand. "It was very nice. I saw some light." *Good-bye,* I thought. *I'm glad I tried it. It was an interesting experience.*

The teacher took my hand in his and seemed to be looking straight into my heart. "There is so much more," he said encouragingly, as if in reply to my internal dialogue. "So much more."

"Can I work in your restaurant in exchange for yoga classes?" I mentally kicked myself. *What in the world am I saying? Oh, well.*

A few weeks won't hurt. I don't have anything better to do. It might be interesting to experience a few more classes.

Walt looked into my eyes with what I can only describe as endless love. Once again he took my hand in his and said, "Welcome home."

CHAPTER 5

THE KARMIC KITCHEN

"Pure foods are those prepared and served in thankful, joyous, kindly loving nature by a person clean in body, sincere in mind, and harmoniously cheerful in character."
—WALT BAPTISTE

*E*veryone ate at the Hungry Mouth: Jerry Garcia, the Jefferson Starship, dancers from the San Francisco Ballet, students and faculty from UCSF Medical Center, and anyone who enjoyed natural fare, lovingly prepared. As one of San Francisco's few authentic health food restaurants of the era, the establishment was always full and had an army of diehard regulars. They came again and again for dishes simple or exotic, from Indian lentils and Aztec-Mayan dishes to Hawaiian prawns with pineapple curry and Egyptian lamb stew over brown rice. Some ate the same thing day after day; some sampled the menu with abandon and delight. For many, the eatery became a home away from home. For me, it was to become even more—a place where I would learn not just about food but about true nourishment of body and soul, about the healing powers of nutrition, and about the karmic meaning of service offered not only with a smile, but with a sincere measure of joy.

But I did not know any of this on the morning I arrived for my first shift. I was nervously thinking about the cigarettes in my purse, wondering how I was going to swing smoking without freaking out the yoga-infused staff.

The day before, after Walt had agreed to let me work in exchange for my classes, I'd left the Center on a cloud. I was catapulted into a state of awareness that was completely new to me. I found myself walking the city's roller coaster streets with a heightened sense of inner composure and self-confidence that was strong and clear. I felt unusually energized and excited beyond words and could think of nothing else other than my extraordinary experience at the yoga center and my meeting with this intriguing and powerful man. It was clear that his students held Walt Baptiste in great esteem, and I was respectful of this reverence, but I had no intention of becoming a member of his group of devoted followers. At the same time, I knew in my gut that I had something momentous to learn from him and I was willing to give myself to this new adventure—at least for the "few weeks" I planned to stick around.

That morning was a reality check. What would my new job be like? Did I have the stuff to do it? I'd never been a waitress before, but I'd grown up in a household where family dinnertime was an inviolable ritual. Each of us seven children was regularly assigned weekly tasks around the cooking, serving, and cleanup of meals. I was no stranger to so-called health food. My parents were whole-grain enthusiasts in the decades when all our neighbors stocked their pantries with Wonder Bread and their refrigerators with soda pop. Sure, I'd had my high school fling with French fries and gravy (every day for lunch, for years), but fruits and vegetables were, so to speak, in my blood. I'd do all right at the Hungry Mouth, wouldn't I? I mean, how hard could it be?

In front of me, the Walt and Magaña Baptiste Yoga and Dance Center loomed. It was a large, four-story art deco building that took up half a city block. Originally, the building was a Masonic temple, which accounted for its massive and ornately designed exterior. The ground level housed a health food store, the Hungry Mouth Restaurant, and Bazaar Boutique, run by Walt's wife, Magaña. All three businesses were connected inside, with the restaurant in the center space. On the second floor were a greeting area, dressing rooms, the meditation room, and the Baptiste gym. The third floor housed a mirrored and colorful dance studio and a large serving kitchen.

The building was situated on one of San Francisco's windiest corners, and as I approached it I noticed Norman, the man who'd served me carrot juice and encouraged me to talk to Walt about working here, diligently sweeping leaves and bits of paper wrappers from outside its doorway. Norman broke his monk-like concentration for a moment to flash me a smile, and I took that as a good omen. Inside, I was directed to Laura, the manager, an attractive thirtyish blonde with a radiant smile, piercing blue eyes, and a perfect figure that I'd soon learn was the result of her own yoga practice, her dance classes with Magaña, and her workouts in the weight gym.

Laura sat down with me in a corner of the dining room—a vibrant space bedecked with Indian paintings, Afghani tapestry, South American wall hangings, and beaded curtains separating the restaurant from the health food store—to work out my schedule. She was businesslike and efficient, but kind. She made it clear that my work hours would be designed to accommodate my attendance at Walt's four weekly yoga classes, and I thought this was very big of her, indeed. I was even more impressed when Laura calmly accepted my query about where I could light up during breaks. "Oh, just step outside," she said matter-of-factly. "The back garden is reserved for meditation, though." I followed her out a private door into a sheltered outdoor area filled with carefully tended potted plants and three individual meditation spaces. Each roofed space had its own bench and was protected on three sides with bamboo fencing.

When it came to my smoking, neither Laura nor anyone else at the restaurant, I soon learned, was prepared to force me to change my wanton ways if I wasn't ready. They were all experienced "karma yogis" who understood that each of us must walk our own path in our own way. But as live-and-let-live as Laura was about personal peccadilloes, when it came to the smooth functioning of the restaurant there were firm rules—and lots of them. Each rule was grounded in what I would come to learn was Walt's carefully thought-out philosophy of food, and every one of them functioned on physical, emotional, and spiritual levels. Walt and company knew full well that people who frequent a restaurant, especially on a repeat basis, are hungry for more than a salad or a sandwich—no matter how savory. They are there, whether they consciously know it or not, for nurturing of a deeper sort.

Laura instructed me in the practical art of waiting tables. She taught me how to recite the list of daily specials, how to speedily convey each order to the kitchen, and how and when to present the check. She painstakingly detailed bussing protocols, stressing that each time diners left a table "it must instantly be made new." But more important than all of that was her intense concern with how I would welcome our customers. "We want everyone to feel at home and glad to be here, so we greet everyone with thankfulness, attentiveness, and cheerfulness," she said. As I was soon to find out, she did in fact mean everyone—even customers who were rude, inconsiderate, or testy; even those we knew would take forever to make up their minds about their orders; even the guy who would invariably come in five minutes before closing time and order the Aztec-Mayan Platter, an entrée featuring spiced corn and plantains that always had to be cooked from scratch. It was our Karma Yoga—the yoga of service—to greet them sincerely, to graciously serve them all, and to find it within ourselves to interact with them from the heart. What came out of our mouths was, apparently, as important as what went into theirs.

Laura was anything but alone in her dedication to viewing the Hungry Mouth as a continual opportunity to practice soup-to-nuts yogic principles. Behind the scenes, above the stove and sinks, behind the cash register, and everywhere the staff was likely to look, signs posted on the walls reminded the waitstaff and chefs of what Walt considered the true intent of our work.

> *Be aware of what you think while you cook.*
> *Your nature is an ingredient in the pots and plates.*
> *Food has a chemical effect and a karmic result.*

The idea that someone's thoughts and attitudes went into a dish along with the salt was something I'd never considered—though I guessed it explained the devotion so many of us feel toward our mothers' love-infused tuna casseroles. But it was clear to me that everyone who worked at the restaurant strove quite earnestly to manifest positive energy as they went about the washing, chopping, preparing, and presenting of breakfast, lunch, and dinner.

The physical work of waiting tables was exhausting. Newly respectful of this craft, I realized it would be demanding to waitress anywhere. But the level of equanimity and concentration expected at the Hungry Mouth was a special challenge for me. In my first weeks at the Center, Walt's yoga classes were having a profound effect on my mindset. I had always been sensitive to the emotions of others. As a child, I was sometimes so empathic that I could not quite tell where other people's feelings left off and mine began. I thought I'd gotten this over-sensitivity under control, but the classes were opening me up in ways I hadn't figured out how to handle yet. I had a new influx of energy into what Walt called the "third eye," and I sometimes felt I could practically read the customers' minds. Along with this, my hearing had mysteriously achieved what felt like "superwoman" powers. I could hear even mumbled conversations on the other side of the crowded room, as if I were sitting right in the customers' laps. Multiply this level of input by all the people I served—each with his or her own personalities and peeves, food-related and otherwise—and it made for a long day.

Out front, Laura kept a watchful eye on me. If I seemed frazzled or lethargic, she would send me to take a break and regroup. Out back, one of the chefs, British-born Colin, took it upon himself to mentor me in the ways of the karmic kitchen. One day, Colin found me self-pityingly scrutinizing a sign above the potato-scrubbing station that said, "A good cook never indulges in self-pity." He came up behind me, put a hand on my shoulder and said softly, "You don't have to be perfect. You just have to be." This Yoda-like exhortation, delivered with Prince Charles diction, somehow left me almost giddy with relief. As if to keep my change of mood going, Colin, a lanky, bespectacled, self-described geek, whose boyish looks belied his forty years, handed me another sort of tonic: a cup of Baptiste Blend Tea. "Two parts peppermint, for the digestion," Colin expounded, "one part alfalfa, for the joints, and one part silica, for the complexion." It was an instant pick-me-up that tasted immensely better than it sounded.

Over the coming months we'd drink quarts of tea a day as Colin answered my many questions about Walt's philosophy of food as an integral part of the yogic path. As I soon learned, Colin held a PhD in physics, but he was now far more concerned with metaphysics, and he and his wife, who worked in the Center's clothing boutique, were two of Walt's longtime students. Colin's spiritual acolyte status and his academic credentials would have been enough to restrain me from asking anything, but he was so down-to-earth and approachable that I came to think of him as the super-smart kid in science class who, if you sat next to him long enough, you realized was just dying to help you out and get you as excited about the periodic table of elements as he was.

"As you grow physically stronger through the yoga practices, the right food chemistry will help build your body," Colin told me. "And as you grow spiritually through meditation, your sensitivity to food increases. The nervous system actually becomes more refined and your psychic abilities sharpen. It's subtle but it's powerful. The right diet supports the shifts but keeps you grounded."

Today, scientific research in the area of nutrition is continually finding correlations between food and specific neurotransmitters in the brain responsible for mood and energy levels. But many decades before most Americans began to even consider the link between food and overall well-being, Colin explained that there was food and then there was *real food*: extraordinary, high-quality sustenance that energizes and uplifts us.

"Pure foods are as close as possible to Mother Nature," said

Colin. "Impure foods are *de*natured, demineralized, devitamin-
ized, and overcooked. When you apply too much fire to food,
even good food, you burn the benefit right out of it. Raw,
uncooked foods contain *prana*."

"What's *prana*?" I asked.

"*Prana* is the yogic equivalent to what the Chinese call *chi*, as
in *t'ai chi*. It's the vital life force. It permeates the universe. Without it, you would be an inanimate object. The more *prana* you
can absorb into your system, the greater energy that you have."

"So . . . no more French fries," I joked.

"Walt says fast foods are made to tease and tempt the appetites of ignorance."

Okay then, I guess not.

"But," he cautioned me, "never forget the 80–20 rule."

Uh-oh, I thought, *another rule*.

"Walt subscribes to the 80–20 theory. If 80 percent of everything that you eat is good for you, then you can have fun foods
for the other 20 percent and your body will be healthy enough
to handle it. It's just when you get the percentages skewed that
you get into trouble."

Now that was a philosophy I could get behind.

The physicist in Colin sometimes emerged when he spoke
about nutrition. According to physics, he said, everything in
this universe is vibration. The physical body that we can see
and feel is a highly refined organism composed of atomic structures vibrating at high rates of speed. Essentially, we're bodies of
energy affected by and affecting everything in our environment.
The foods we take into our bodies also have differing vibrational
frequencies. Higher-frequency foods like uncooked fruits, vegetables, sprouted grains, seeds, and nuts, are rich in enzymes
and life force, and contribute to vitality. Lower-frequency foods

like processed and chemically altered foods, are a drain on our energetic system. The body has to expend tremendous effort to transform and eliminate them.

As for the link between food and thought, Colin explained that since thoughts are also vibrations, our thoughts and attitudes during eating have a profound effect on digestion as well as on our more subtle energetic body. And when we eat food prepared by others, we take into ourselves the consciousness and quality of thoughts held by the person preparing the food. Even the intention of the people who grow the food has a subtle influence on what we eat. Suddenly, it made perfect sense to me that the thoughts and feelings we in the kitchen held while preparing food for our customers impacted their whole beings.

When it came to preparing pure food, Baptiste style, Colin walked the walk. His work style was a wonder to watch, exemplifying Walt's maxim that "one can be sloppy or thoughtful in the same measure of time." Colin could slice and dice more quickly and precisely than the most effusive late-night infomercial knife hawker, but no matter what, he'd always give the essential ingredients enough time to bring out the intrinsic flavors of a dish. For Colin, preparing each plate even more perfectly than he did the time before was more than a habit or a point of professional pride: it was a true yogic practice.

The other eight yoga students working in the restaurant—most of them males—were equally colorful characters with fascinating backgrounds. Jon, a former naval officer who served in Vietnam, was also an accomplished classical pianist. His humor and energy levels were off the charts, and he prided himself on being down to earth. Anytime I started to get too "wooey-wooey" for his taste he would say, "Don't give me any of that metaphysical claptrap." He said I had a great heart and he fondly called me "Lovey."

Head chef Matthew was the coworker with whom I became friendliest. Just a few years older than I, and a fellow Midwesterner that I instantly related to, he occasionally invited me to hop on his motorcycle after work and head to North Beach for some local San Francisco nightlife and a chat over some brews.

I used the opportunity to satisfy my curiosity about parts of Walt's life I knew little about.

"So what's with the Baptiste kids?" I asked him at the first opportunity. Walt and Magaña had three children, who were always in and out of the Center. "What an unusual lifestyle to be brought up in," I said, remembering my far more conventional upbringing.

Matthew explained that Sherri, the oldest Baptiste daughter, actually owned the health food store. I knew she was a few years younger than I and this impressed me to no end. I couldn't imagine myself taking on that kind of responsibility, or wanting to. But Sherri seemed up to the job, and even at her young age her presence was warm and nurturing beyond her years.

Devi Ananda Baptiste, then in her late teens, was the younger of the two daughters. I had seen her in a belly dancing performance and was mesmerized by her exquisite grace and beauty. Several hours a week, she worked in Magaña's boutique, where her peals of laughter could often be heard throughout the Center. The youngest Baptiste was a ten-year-old boy, Baron. He was a high-energy kid with a sunny disposition who was usually decked out in a Chinese kung fu suit and slippers.

"Everyone at the center has their own unique relationship with Walt," said Matthew as he poured himself a cold one. "His children know that they are held in a special way. Walt makes that very clear to all of us. But since they were small, those kids have been raised surrounded by us students. They treat us as part of their larger spiritual family."

During one of our evening sojourns, I shared with Matthew my confusion about the guru-disciple relationship, which many of the students seem to have with Walt, and where I fit into the picture. "I don't get it, Matthew. Everyone seems to tiptoe around Walt, and at the same time they adore him. Sometimes he's so loving, and other times he's so strict. What's going on?"

"It's not that black and white, Michele. There are things operating at the Center that are far deeper than the obvious. By now you must be aware of that. You don't just simply stumble across Walt Baptiste and his teachings. It's your karma that brought you here."

"What about the guru thing?" I asked. Why do some students call him Walt and others call him *Gurudev*?" I certainly had no intention of being a guru's disciple and had never had the slightest inkling from Walt that he expected it.

"Look, Michele, there are gurus in every culture, on every continent, and in every wisdom tradition. You could easily replace the word *guru* with *shaman, high priest,* and *priestess,* or even *medicine man.* Unfortunately, in the West, because of a few questionable characters, the term has gotten a bad rap, but in India it is a highly respected title bestowed upon spiritual teachers.

"You have to retrace the origin of the meaning of the word *guru*," Matthew said. "It means 'dispeller of darkness' or 'one who leads from darkness to light.' A guru is a spiritual teacher who has been through all of the tests of this world and is showing us how to break through our dense subconscious conditioning. He's not really interested in whether we like him or not. It's his job to take us to the next step, and he knows exactly what to do to help us get there."

"But I don't even know what step I'm on right now, or what to expect next. All I know is that for some strange reason, it's really important for me to listen to Walt's guidance. Sometimes he seems to know exactly what I'm thinking and feeling. Maybe that ought to scare me, but I'm happier than I've ever been." I hesitated before adding, "The restaurant is tough, though. I'm learning a lot, but I've never worked so hard in my life!"

Matthew smiled knowingly. "It gets better and better, Michele. Hang in there. It's totally worth it." As if to punctuate the discussion, he poured himself another beer.

❧

It turned out Matthew's prediction was correct. In a very short time, I was swept up in the joy and camaraderie of life at the Center. At the restaurant, the pleasures of the kinship began to outweigh the trials of the actual labor. To make matters even better, I was now being paid in cash as well as trading waitressing duties for yoga classes.

Sometimes on my work breaks, when the restaurant was empty and the guys were in the kitchen making preparations for dinner, I would sneak into the health food store and talk to Norman.

I still lovingly refer to Norman as the yoga center's resident Chinese sage. Born in Hawaii, Norman spoke with a blend of erudite English and pidgin Hawaiian slang—just enough of the latter to soften his potentially daunting intellect. Norman was a walking encyclopedia of knowledge on almost any subject you could name. His delivery always had the ring of absolute certainty. He had an air of ultimate credibility in whatever subject he was discussing at the moment. The curious thing about him is that not only was he infinitely knowledgeable about the spiritual path, but he was equally savvy about things like sports, and could recite baseball card details from the 1950s that would overload my mind. Then, in the next sentence, as he stood behind the counter in the health food store, he would expound on the healing properties of French green clay.

I learned Norman had a master's in English literature and had taught English on the island of Molokai before coming to San Francisco, but apart from this, he was a consummate autodidact. He would become intrigued with a topic and research everything there was to know about it. He did this the old-fashioned way, cloistering himself in university libraries, for this was long before the age of Google and Wikipedia.

Norman had been a Baptiste student longer than anyone else at the Center and was a friend and counselor to all. He selflessly helped us all to the degree that we needed it. I had no idea how old he was. I only knew that he was older than me—and infinitely wiser. In the gym, he bench-pressed his own weight without the use of a rack, a bodybuilding feat of which not many can boast, and was a master teacher of the mind–body relationship long before it became the trend.

Norm was a permanent fixture at the Baptiste Center and literally lived in the rafters of the building. I never actually saw his space—only the stairway leading from the doorway off the third floor dance studio up to his mysterious inner sanctum, where I imagined him in deep meditation from night until daybreak.

I wasn't the only student who held Norman in great esteem. Despite the occasional spiritual sibling rivalry or differences among the students at the center at any given time (after all, we were a family, and what family doesn't have occasional squabbles?), there was one issue that we all firmly agreed upon. That was unconditional love and gratitude for Norman.

Norman was the middleman of Walt Baptiste's teachings, and during my first two years at the Center I was happily under his tutelage. He loved to discuss the big spiritual picture, and did so with a matter-of-fact delivery that was grounded but ethereal. In response to my mundane complaints and litanies of personal difficulties, Norman would remind me of my higher purpose and lift me out of my "woe is me" attitude. Echoing my earlier discussion with Matthew, Norman assured me, "This is an esoteric school of higher learning. It's no accident that you're here. You've earned it from your previous work with the teacher in past lifetimes."

Soon enough, despite the fact that no one at the Hungry Mouth pressured me to do so, I decided to quit smoking. Whether it was the effect of my yoga classes, my new vegetarian diet, or of the weight-training regime I'd now also added to my schedule, I'm not sure. But it was time. I entered a behavioral training program called Smoke No Longer, the idea behind which was to make smoking so unpleasant, so inconvenient, and so downright gross that you'd almost beg someone to take your cigarettes away. After four weeks of storing my butts in a jar of rapidly blackening water and engaging in other such nauseating techniques, the mere thought of lighting up sent a shiver down my yogicly straightened spine. Once I'd quit, I felt a powerful urge to get years of toxins out of my system. Under

Norman's guidance, I went on a three-day juice fast, which left me feeling clear and renewed. In fact, I was astonished at how much better and lighter I felt, both physically and mentally. The initial experience of feeling the effects of diet on my thinking and emotional state left an indelible impression on me. Over the coming years, I'd read voraciously and experiment with raw foods, macrobiotics, and other dietary regimes, to personally experience what each system gave back. I discovered that each system of eating creates its own consciousness, energy, and healing qualities, and that each had its place at different periods of my life.

My quitting smoking should have had one additional benefit that, in fact, did not manifest as quickly as I thought it might. My need to light up had been my excuse for coming back late from restaurant breaks on occasion. But now it seemed that, smoking or no smoking, I *still* tended to be a little late coming back from breaks. I now chalked this up to my being a "free spirit" at heart, but this lack of punctuality did not meet the high standards set by my colleagues. Then one day, something very strange happened that led me to change my tardy ways.

I'd been given a free ticket to the American Conservatory Theater to see a two o'clock matinee. I was excited about going and figured that if I asked to move my usual lunch break and timed everything just right, I could pull it off. The chefs razzed me, at once teasing and serious, that I'd mess up my karma if I didn't make it back at the start of my shift. It turned out the play went longer than I thought, and the bus I boarded back to the restaurant was crowded and made every stop. I searched desperately through my purse for a quarter so I could jump off and at least make a phone call explaining my whereabouts, but all I had was a dime. I skulked into the kitchen fifteen minutes past my deadline. The chefs hardly talked to me. Suddenly, in walked Walt. He smiled at me with an impish and loving grin. Then, he pulled a quarter out of his pocket.

"Were you looking for this?" he said.

Clearly, there was more going on here than met the eye.

CHAPTER 6

LIFTING

"Develop the body to its highest in every way as natural law will allow. For in beauty, strength, health, when a body exists as such, its possessor is an artist who has done a work well. The mind then is allowed greater expansion because of its improved physical instrument."

—WALT BAPTISTE

Walt Baptiste's telepathic ability was, apparently, well known to the longtime students at the Center. It was more or less assumed by everyone that he had a way of intuiting what you'd been up to, and virtually everyone had stories to tell about how he'd spoken to them "out of the blue" about goings-on of which he'd had no material means of knowing. At first, I chalked up his uncanny knack to keen observational skills and coincidence. But Walt's allusions to things that had happened to me a day or a week before or, on occasion, as far back as childhood, became a frequent occurrence.

One day, I was clearly daydreaming when I was supposed to be on duty, and Walt commented that I was "doodling lotuses in my head." The lotus, I'd found out only recently, was the name of the flower whose image I'd drawn obsessively in grade school when I was supposed to be listening to the sisters. How could he have known what I'd never known myself until days before and never mentioned to a soul? And why did he want to know? I began to wonder if for some reason Walt was keeping a kind of karmic report card. Maybe I'd better start listening even more closely to what he was trying to tell me.

Another day, he came into the restaurant while I was in the midst of a defensive meltdown in response to one of my co-workers criticizing my questionable vacuuming technique. When I saw him enter, I immediately shifted my defensive internal muttering and began repeating *Peace, harmony, well-being*. Walt's eyes met mine and he said, "Thank you." My inner jaw dropped. *Oh my god*, I thought. *He really does know what I'm thinking*.

And so it went one morning when I was in the process of quitting smoking. Worried about my slowing metabolism and possible flabby results, I'd awakened early, done a bunch of sit-ups and as many push-ups as I could manage, then ran around Golden Gate Park until I got a side stitch. I'd had to sit recovering on a bench for twenty minutes before I could limp home. Later that day, after yoga class, Walt came over to me and said in his prescient way, "If you're interested in shaping up, forget mindless exercise; you need mindful exercise. I suggest you start going to the gym."

Aargh, I thought, *the gym. I guess I should have known this was coming.*

The weight training gym was an integral part of the Baptistes' holistic complex. Among his many accomplishments, Walt was a bodybuilding champion—a former Mr. America—and the founding editor of *Body Moderne*, a weight-lifting and health-oriented magazine published from the late forties to the early fifties. Though he was fifty-six when I met him, both he and Magaña (who was an erstwhile Miss Universe runner-up), were phenomenal examples of strength, vitality, and radiant health. Magaña, a dark-eyed Latin beauty with a cascade of jet-black shoulder-length hair, had the dynamic personality of a triple Leo—outgoing and vivacious. I learned through the Center's grapevine that Walt had one of the first gyms in the U.S. to allow women, and that Magaña was a pioneer in the U.S. as both a female yoga teacher and in cultivating and teaching the art of physical culture.

Located on the second floor of the building, the red-carpeted weight room had a salon feel and an overall décor that was meant to be cozy and inviting—though it was not so, at this point, to me. The gym's threshold had a carved wooden sign above the door inscribed with the words GOOD★TRUTH★BEAUTY. But when I first encountered it, all I could think was NOT★FOR★ME. I was certain that the gym just wasn't, as we said in the seventies, my thing. In fact, it seemed the very opposite of what I was interested in. My interest was a higher state of consciousness. What could lifting barbells possibly have to do with that?

I tried to ignore Walt's suggestion for a week or two. But the teacher's suggestions, as it turned out, were not to be ignored. In fact, they weren't suggestions; they were more like road signs you had to follow if you didn't want to go around in circles. One day in yoga class, he looked straight at me and stated his point of view a bit more forcefully. "The gym is not optional on this path," he said. I stifled a sigh, and Walt smiled.

The next morning, I folded some tights and a leotard into a paper bag and arrived at the Center an hour before my morning shift at the restaurant. Norman, as usual, was outside sweeping (what time did he start?), but he turned to me and said, "Go on up. I'll be right there."

A bright young woman with sparkling blue eyes and long, wavy, reddish-brown hair warmly greeted me at the gym's front desk. "You must be Michele. I'm Sandra." Her small and compact frame and her classic black leotard and exotic-looking fuchsia harem pants lent an air of femininity to what I perceived as a male-dominated gym atmosphere. It seemed Sandra also worked in the upstairs area, teaching yoga, dance, and weight lifting.

"Have you been working out in the gym a long time?" I casually asked her.

"Oh, yes," she said cheerily. "I've been working for the Baptistes for twelve years and began using the gym shortly after starting yoga. Norm says he's working with you this morning. He'll be right up."

She turned to answer the phone and waved me into the gym.

In addition to his work in the health food store, his shifts at the yoga studio's front desk, and his perennial broom wielding, Norman served as one of three primary gym instructors/yoga teachers—the others being Sandra and Big John, a six-foot-six gentle giant. They were de facto personal trainers long before personal training became a popular profession. Apparently, Norm had more to teach me in yet another area.

Waiting for Norman to come upstairs, I surveyed what I could only think of as the instruments of torture that were about to be unleashed upon me. There were free weights and barbells of all sizes, a leg press machine that required lying on your back and pressing straight up, a quadriceps raise, several slant boards, and a foot roller. Strategically placed above the foot roller was a four- by five-foot sign meant to be at eye level while you sat and massaged your soles. It quoted Plato: "The happiest man is he who most feels that he is improving himself—the best man is

he who most improves himself." Adorning the walls were post-
ers and photos of Walt and Magaña in their bodybuilding days,
along with many signed photos and notes from bodybuilding
champions who had trained with them in the 1940s, '50s, and
'60s. I skimmed through some of the notes and saw that many
alluded to Walt's unique method of using the mind and incor-
porating visualization to help change the body. From the looks
of the bodybuilders' physiques, his methods must have been
exceptionally successful.

I was eying my own thimble-sized biceps when Norman
arrived. He must have read my mind—there seemed to be a
lot of this going around—because the first thing he said to me
was, "Michele, I know what you're interested in, so I'm going
to explain all this to you in a way that will make 'spiritual sense.'
Walt believes in the philosophy of working from a strong base
upward. The work you do in the gym will give you a strong
foundation from which to grow. This will keep you grounded
as you dive into the subtler meditation practices."

He looked me up and down, carefully sizing up the task at
hand.

"I'll give you a workout regime, and that's going to change
every six weeks so your body won't have a chance to adapt and
get lazy. But there are certain things that will never change. And
those are the most important things."

Norman went on to tell me that what went on in the gym
was actually a form of yoga, that progressive weight training
was yet another means of anchoring myself to the moment—of
being fully present and of growing in every aspect of being. He
then launched into an explanation of correct breathing while I
fidgeted, impatient to begin exercising. Then, it struck me that
this was the way my father had taught his beginning flutists.

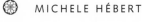

He did not have them pick up the flute until the very end of their first lesson. "The foundation of any wind instrument," my father would explain, "is mastery of the breath."

I started listening to Norman more closely.

"The weights strengthen the physical body but also balance the emotional body," Norman said. "The breathing you do when you lift the weight draws in *prana*"—there was that word again—"and that balances your physical energies, which correspond to your mental and emotional body processes."

This was a concept I had never considered. "Do you mean that when I strengthen one part of myself the other parts are also affected?"

"Well, not exactly. Your question assumes that they are separate bodies when, actually, mind and body are one. A conscious shift in one automatically equals a shift in the other. The key is concentration. You become the sculptor of your body-mind vehicle, molding and shaping it into the form that you desire, and this extends out into your life.

"You work with the weights and the weights work with you," Norman went on. "The heavier the weight, the more it pulls your mind into the muscle. That's what makes the body develop. Two people can do the same routine, eat the same diet, but if one progresses more, it's often because of their level of concentration on the part of the body they are working."

This metaphysical approach to physical strength got my attention, and I agreed to let Norman design an introductory program for me. He demonstrated a basic routine of twelve exercises that evenly addressed all the major muscle groups. It looked simple enough—as it should have been for Norman, who could bench press his own weight—but I found it harder to execute than I'd imagined. Even though the weights were light, I was flailing, and I felt completely uncoordinated. The reason, Norman assured me, was not that I was a hopeless weakling or an inveterate klutz, but that I was alternating between holding my breath and huffing and puffing.

"In the gym, we want to increase your breathing capacity," Norman said. "Breath is life, and we want to draw more life force into the system. As you gracefully coordinate lifting and breathing, you'll increase your chest capacity and your pranic energy levels."

"But I already know how to breathe," I protested. I'd been doing it since the moment I was born. Nothing to it.

"Yes," he responded patiently, "but you have a habit of breathing that keeps you at a certain level, physically and mentally. It's intertwined with your habits of thinking and your emotional reactions. When you learn to breathe more fully, you will also expand your mind and your perceptions of life. And it will help you in your meditation practice. It's all related."

He went on to explain further. "As a yogi, you want to increase your ability to take in *prana*. The problem is that you can only take in as much air as you have room to breathe."

"So how do I do that if my lung capacity is already set?"

"You make more room from the inside out by breathing more deeply than you normally do. Look," he went on, "the standard breathing instruction in weight lifting is to exhale on the exertion. But it's so much more than that. It's the quality of attention on the breath that matters. You want the breath to motivate the muscle to move the weight."

"So, my breath moves the weight and not the muscle?" This was getting more interesting.

"Exactly. A yogi rides the breath flow in the gym and in life. But breath awareness and capacity are key. When you inhale, your chest doesn't simply open to the front. As human beings, we have the ability to breathe to the sides of the lungs and the back of the lungs. But most people have never even considered breathing to the back of their lungs."

No kidding, I thought.

"If you are highly aware of the breath, you fill out the muscles in between the ribs to increase capacity. You see some people lifting heavy weights and they're just not breathing with the right intent, even in heavy bench presses. They're putting muscle on top of their chest, not expanding it from the inside. It's an entirely different result in consciousness and in the shape their body takes."

Over the next few weeks, I began to feel more comfortable in my workouts. My muscles became more flexible, my movements more graceful. I learned to understand my body not just as a physical vehicle but also as a reflection of my mental state. I noticed that every time I felt stuck in the gym, there was an emotional place that needed to be unstuck. I began to tame the negative states of mind that worked against me as I worked out. If I hated lunges—which I did, with a passion—I tried thinking joyful thoughts as I did them, and soon, the exercise was hateful no more. I was literally reprogramming myself.

Overall, I felt stronger and more energetic, which was all the better for my yoga practice, not to mention for the work of carrying heaping plates down at the Hungry Mouth. But what I gained went beyond that—the lifting helped me practice feeling grounded in the moment; the full and complete breathing it required deepened my meditation practice and helped to purify my cluttered mind.

I speak from firsthand experience when I say that mental purification is a major player on the spiritual path, any spiritual path. I was constantly being reminded everywhere I turned that once we step onto the path of self-mastery, the weaker part of ourselves that doesn't want to change starts yelling and screaming with all its might to keep us from progressing. A mighty battle ensues on a mental and emotional level that is not for the faint of heart. I found myself in a daily struggle to get hold of my unpredictable mind, and sometimes felt as if I was losing it altogether.

"You're not alone," Norman reminded me. "Every spiritual aspirant goes through the process of purification. It's part of the game. If you really want to progress on this path, you have to face your weaknesses and clear them out as they surface. That's the story of Ulysses and the Sirens. That's the story of Perseus and Medusa. It's knights versus dragons. The demons are never really outer demons. They represent our own demons lying beneath the surface. You are readying yourself for great work ahead. It's not easy, Michele. But the payoff is big. And here you are being supported and given the tools to get through it in one piece. The gym is one of those tools. Use it well."

And use it I did, with great enthusiasm—especially when, after the first three weeks, I clearly saw my body changing and felt more graceful and self-assured in my workout routine. At first, I went to the gym almost daily, even though the recommended schedule was three days a week. I would walk into the gym out of whack and off balance mentally and emotionally, and leave balanced and happy. And always there was Norman, a steady and dependable reminder of my real purpose in it all.

Now I had a glimmer of the big picture here at the Center. Everything was related to everything. At its essence, this was a university of consciousness with a vast interdisciplinary curriculum. Each advancement freed you to delve deeper, climb higher.

As the gym became a regular part of my life, I also got to know more of the Center "regulars." I learned that Walt had been a pioneer and champion in the early days of bodybuilding. He was one of the first to emphasize the use of the mind in changing the body's musculature and an early advocate of nutrition and breathing in sculpting the body. He also was the first to sing "Somewhere over the Rainbow," when he won a Mr. America bodybuilding contest. Walt, it turned out, possessed a highly developed sense of whimsy along with his other gifts.

Swapping Walt stories was a favorite pastime as we rested between sets or packed up our gear. I learned that Walt had been a pioneer and champion in the early days of bodybuilding. He was one of the first to emphasize the use of the mind in changing the body's musculature and an early advocate of nutrition and breathing in sculpting the body. He was also the first to sing "Somewhere over the Rainbow" when he won a championship bodybuilding contest. Walt, it turned out, possessed a highly developed sense of whimsy along with his other gifts.

As at the Hungry Mouth, everybody at the gym had a story about Walt. But some were better than others. One day, I was strolling out of the gym beside a muscular young man I thought of as "motorcycle guy" because he always arrived at the center on a giant Harley. I shared with him my anecdote about Walt's somehow knowing I'd needed a quarter that day I was late coming back from the theater.

"That's nothing," he said. "One night about five years ago, I was in a fight outside a bar in Milwaukee where I was living, and this guy pulled out a gun, aimed it at my chest, and shot me.

At the moment the gun went off, I saw a man's body—well, the face and shape of a man's body, but made out of light—fly between me and the bullet. Later, at the hospital, the doctors said that bullet stopped millimeters from my spine without penetrating it. They called it a miracle. About two years ago, I moved to San Francisco, came here to the Center, and met Walt. I recognized him right away. He was the man made out of light."

CHAPTER 7

PRACTICE, PRACTICE, PRACTICE

"Lead me from the unreal to the real. Lead me from dark-
ness to light. Lead me from death to immortality."
—UPANISHADS

orking at the Hungry Mouth and working out at the
gym were physical enterprises of the most earthbound sort. My
feet could attest to this by the way they ached after a long
day waiting tables, and my muscles from the way they gratefully responded to a warm bath after I'd added more weights
to my training routine. Yet, both these activities tapped continually into a more transcendent energy, and I came to see
them for what they were: a part of my deepening yoga practice.
Nowhere, however, did this energy manifest more intensely
than in Walt's four weekly yoga classes, which I made it my top
priority to attend.

The day I sampled my first class I was conscious—or rather,
I was *self*-conscious—of my novice status. There were students
who had been with Walt for years. I wondered if I shouldn't be
in some kind of beginner's class. But Walt said, "There are no
beginners on the yogic path. Everyone is on a spiritual journey
from the moment you are born, and when you've learned all

you could from a given situation, life promotes you." In each class, you were exactly where you were supposed to be, and your job was to make progress.

Many yoga students think of progress in yoga as perfecting their headstand or finally managing not to tip over in crow pose. But this is not what Walt meant. Walt Baptiste was a master of Raja Yoga, or the royal yoga. Raja Yoga is nothing less than a blueprint for living life, a path of discovering universal principles. As Walt said, it is a system that was "designed for the purposeful evolution of consciousness." Raja Yoga encompasses the eight limbs of yoga originating five thousand years ago and set forth two thousand years ago by the Hindu sage Patanjali, author of the *Yoga Sutras*. It includes meditative practices, devotional practices, Karma Yoga—that is, the yoga of selfless service—and Hatha Yoga, which is the practice of physical postures or *asanas*. There's a lot to be gained from a good Hatha Yoga class—indeed, Magaña taught a dynamic and colorful one interspersed with inspirational readings (and she still does so at age eighty-nine), but Walt's approach was unique. He used *asanas* not as ends in themselves, but rather as means to greater ends.

In a typical sixty-minute class, we students might assume five or six postures, holding each for ten or twelve minutes. At first, each pose might have felt easy, a cakewalk. *I can do this forever, no sweat!* But soon they grew challenging, and eternity itself seemed to loom mockingly. *Yeah, girl, you can do this for how long?* But Walt guided us through our difficulties. He had us maintain steady, conscious nostril breaths and direct each breath more deeply into the area being opened. Once we truly settled, all physical discomfort gone and the mind no longer running wild, it felt as though we were born in that particular position, and would be happy to stay in it until the sun went supernova. While we first suffered in and then relaxed fully into forward bends or knee-to-chest poses, Walt would speak to us in words that were meant to penetrate our psyches and souls at specific deep levels. Knowing we hold our beliefs not simply in our heads, but in muscle and bone and in the very cell structure of our bodies, Walt would say things to us—sometimes seemingly simple things—that somehow erased years of ingrained fears or negativity that had been running through our subconscious minds like endless loops of bad, yet barely noticeable, Muzak.

While we were in an open and accessible state, Walt would encourage us to let go of blame, past resentments, and revenge. *"Get hold of your mind or negativity will."*

He discouraged us from speaking pessimistically or from spreading gossip and rumor. *"Master the tongue and soon you will master the tongue of the mind."*

He even suggested that we reimagine the way in which we prayed, pointing out that much prayer was not, in fact, communication with the divine, but rather begging and pleading and whining—*please God, give me this; please God, don't give me that.* Why not be receptive to God? Why not listen to God, Walt said, instead of presenting the Almighty with a shopping list?

For me, during those classes it often felt like Walt was reading my thoughts and responding directly to my inner dialogue. If I was frantically wishing I could extricate myself from a pose— *Are we done yet, are we done yet?*—Walt would calmly say, "You think you will move and everything will be alright. The grass is always greener on the other side of the fence. The goal is to be well in what you are doing in this moment."

If I even thought about peeking at how another student was holding a posture so that I could compare myself for better or worse, he would gently chide, "Just do what you are here to do. Stay on your own prayer mat." Everything was grist for the mill, a life lesson. Or rather, a *lives* lesson. I came to understand that Walt was enabling us to cut through many lifetimes' worth of mental and emotional clutter at an accelerated pace. It might not have been instant karma, but it was certainly a sped-up version.

Sometimes, just before class, something would happen that would throw me for a loop. I'd think about not going to yoga, but staying home to sleep, sulk, or stew instead. When I would go after all, Walt would inevitably say something that clarified my problem or turned my perspective on its head. At one point, I had engaged in a romantic dalliance with a man who was already "taken." I arrived in class riddled with guilt and uncertain how to handle the uncomfortable situation I had gotten myself into. But Walt erased any doubt I had when he spent a long time instructing the class on the dangers of tampering with your karma. "There are some people who are meant to be in your life and some who are not," he said. "It is your job to know the difference." He sternly ended, "Don't do this to your karma." Case closed.

One day, I'd been wholly unnerved during a bus ride for reasons I couldn't explain. It was a strange and frightening experience. Everything felt okay when I boarded the bus and was standing next to the driver, but the bus became crowded and I had to move toward the back. I found myself surrounded by many odd-looking people, some of whom appeared to be staring at me with faces that were strangely distorted. It was like a scene from Rod Serling's *The Twilight Zone*. It felt to me like everyone nearby me was either in a state of fear or acute depression. I felt trapped and helpless in the face of this suffering, and a feeling of panic began to rise up inside of me. I tried to tune out the sensations and focus on a tiny portable *Bhagavad-Gita*, the ancient Hindu scripture I carried in my handbag, but it was no use. Finally, after what seemed like an eternity, the bus arrived at my stop and I quickly got off. The incident left me shaken. It was a huge relief to arrive at the tranquility of the yoga center.

Later, when class began, Walt said—very pointedly, I thought—"What is within is without. The mind is like a radio and our minds are like stations on the dial. We vibrate at different frequencies and so pick up different wavelengths of thoughts. But even the most evil thoughts will not penetrate a higher frequency. There is a way of paradise and a way of hell. It is up to you. It is all in your mind."

I instantly understood this to be true. The very receptivity I was cultivating in my practice needed to be tamed and trained. My boundaries were too fluid and there were still parts of myself that could too easily resonate with the negative. Walt was telling me clearly that what I experienced on that bus was nothing less than certain elements of myself I still needed to face, to accept, and to purify.

I left that class feeling like a new door had been opened. I stopped to tell Norman, who was manning the reception desk, about my revelation, but although he smiled beatifically he made no comment. Many years later, Norman told me that after virtually every class, at least half a dozen students would come up to him and tell him that they had experienced an amazing revelation, that it was as if Walt had been speaking primarily to them, that somehow he had managed to give them exactly what they required at the very moment they needed it most.

The funny thing is that each and every one of us was right.

People came to the Center for different reasons. There were

spiritual seekers, to be sure, but there were also those who came to improve their overall health and flexibility, to revel in the joys of the dance, or simply to learn the art of relaxation and take a soothing break from their otherwise hectic days. Everyone received what they sought. Often much more.

About four weeks into my classes I glimpsed something "more." It was not something I was consciously looking for, because it was not something I was aware existed, at least not beyond words.

In every class, Walt Baptiste spoke about Light. I'm capitalizing that *L* because he was not talking about a bulb or a candle or a lantern, or even the light of the sun, moon, or stars. His teachings have been called the Path of Light. Intellectually I knew that the Light he referred to is the source of all things, of life and energy. It is the heart of the soul or, as Kabir wrote, "the breath inside the breath." But the existence of this Light was, for me, merely a comforting concept. It was an idea; it was an aspiration—nothing more. I registered the words, but of experience, I was ignorant.

Then, everything changed.

I was in a pose that had me seated on my heels, spine erect, with my palms face down on my thighs. The real work we were doing in class that day involved a practice of balancing the energies of left and right through ever-so-subtle contractions, beginning with the pressure of the palms into the thighs, and matching this with the entire body evenly in concert with the breath. Suddenly, at the site of my so-called third eye, deep behind the center of my forehead, the Light appeared. The most intense feelings of love, exquisite goodness, bliss, radiance of being, and completion emanated from deep within it and encompassed every part of my being—body, mind, emotions. Every thought and feeling I had ever experienced in my life paled in relation to this divine Light. It was an exquisitely beautiful and powerful force. It was perfect love. Perfection itself. And it was me. I experienced myself as pure radiant Light, not separate from anyone or anything. At that moment, I also realized with absolute certainty that this Light is in every single person—although most of us just don't know it.

As that realization overtook me, I also became aware of something happening in the room. In the distance I could hear, or rather, sense, that Walt had moved from his usual position in front of the class and was standing beside me. His voice was reverberating, and he was whispering passionately *Yes, yes, yes*. I was sure then, absolutely positive, that this was all real. It was more real, in fact, than anything that had ever happened to me before.

Walt stayed with me until the light faded. The class was over and I could hear people leaving, but I did not want to move the tiniest muscle and break the deep awareness of my precious experience. I was filled with a peace beyond measure.

⌁

For the next few days, I walked around in an expansive state of wonder and excitement that gradually transformed into a fever for more Light. I didn't say a word to anyone, but at every opportunity I tried to get it back. I assumed that it would now appear on a daily basis and that all I had to do was show up. No such luck. As hard as I tried and prayed and replayed the exact steps to the inner Light, it remained as elusive as it had the first twenty-six years of my life. After a week, I was confused and miserable.

In class the following Saturday, Walt addressed my spiritual dilemma: "In the Bible, Jesus said, 'Keep thy mind's eye single and thy whole body shall be filled with Light.' We do not ask for blind belief. Through our teachings, you are given firsthand experience of your own inner resource, which is divine Light. But you are like a fifty-watt light bulb. If you shoot ten thousand watts of energy into it, it will explode. You must prepare the vehicle, including the nervous system, to be able to absorb this intensity of spiritual energy."

In the many years since this event, I have found myself hesitant to describe it. One reason is that an experience of such intense power is often best left undiluted and undissected. But another is that I know that whatever I say, words will inevitably fail me. Others who have experienced this divine Light seem only to capture it through poetry or art. Rumi did it best, I think, although Kabir comes close. But how can I compare myself to either of these great mystics? Bob, a fellow Baptiste student and songwriter, described his own experience in a song he called "Light, How I Love Thee." It touches on the incredible feeling a similar experience evoked in him. His music is alive inside of me but, oddly, his words always seem to escape me. I have asked myself over and over how to find my own words. Where are the words adequate to tell what I "know" in my being?

The closest image my mind can fathom on this plane of existence is a dawn one morning on a beach in El Salvador. Before the sun rose to the horizon, it was preceded by the brightest yet most translucent light I had ever seen in this world. I felt that if I held my gaze for too long, its intensity would be blinding. I will never forget its power and majesty as long as I live. Yet even this celestial radiance was a pinpoint compared to the intensity and bliss of the Light I experienced that day in the middle of a "routine" yoga class in a studio in San Francisco.

In a moment, I was forever changed, as was my relationship with Walt. In an instant, he became my guru in the deepest meaning of the word. The Light ignited a fire in my soul—a quest for life's meaning, for my meaning. I yearned to know more. Where had I come from? What is my purpose? Its memory has kept me going whenever I grow weary or skeptical or in any way tuned into those "lower frequencies" on the dial.

One thing I do know is what Walt would say: that each of us must experience such truths for ourselves. No matter how many words rain down upon us, they cannot penetrate our deepest places. To move from darkness to light, from the unreal to the real, there is only one way: "*Practice, practice, practice. Lo—behold the goal!*"

CHAPTER 8

IN TRANSIT

"Each man dies and is being reborn daily. For no man is totally the same today as he was yesterday, or even an hour before."

—WALT BAPTISTE

November 1976

The red-eye from San Francisco took off for El Salvador's international airport right on time. From my vantage point in the rear of the plane, where I was wedged between two fellow travelers from the Center, I could see Walt several rows ahead, sitting with his spine perfectly erect. On my left, Sandra, the capable and calm brunette who for fifteen years had shared front desk duties with Norman, noticed me watching him. "We're like three ducklings following the mother duck," she observed. Then, she scrunched a small requisition airline pillow beneath her neck, hoping to catch a few hours' sleep.

I was honored to be traveling with Sandra, who was now one of the senior teachers at the Center. In addition to her yoga and gym instruction, she was an exceptional teacher of East Indian and Middle Eastern dance. My mind traveled back to my very first belly dancing party at the Center, attended by 135 people in full costume. Sandra was a featured dancer, complete with boa constrictor. Barely five feet tall, she was in complete control as her hips circled, and she undulated to the rhythm of the musical troupe, led by Walt on drums and flute. Her pet snake, Josua, encircled her outstretched arms, holding the audience mesmerized. This was followed by a sword dance in which she performed intricate floor work—belly dancing lingo for acrobatic backbends and other writhing movements on the floor with a huge sword balanced on her body, or on her head—or precariously perched on a foot extending dramatically into the air. The intensity of her concentration had the audience holding its breath in unison, momentarily hypnotized. Instantly, my preconceived notions of Sandra as a quiet, serene, low-key (and, yes, slightly boring) yoga teacher, lay in smithereens at my feet.

On my right during our flight, petite, vivacious Marina, a young woman who'd appeared at the Center shortly after I did, was holding her long, wavy blonde hair back as she pored over one of the many magazines she'd commandeered from the stewardess. Marina was primarily a yoga student of Magaña's and occasionally helped out in the restaurant. She took delight in the absurd and displayed a dry wit that could shift the dourest of moods. Without looking up, she began softly humming the tune to "We're Off to See the Wizard" and glanced at me from the corner of her eye to see if I got it. I rolled my eyes in response.

I was far too excited to nap or read. To occupy my time, and knowing that my guru was in the immediate vicinity, I extracted my *mala* from my backpack, allowing my fingers to touch each of its 108 prayer beads in turns. I began to alternate the mantras that had come to be such an important part of my life over the past two years. One was *peace, harmony, well-being*, the mantra Walt encouraged all his yoga students to use; the other was *joy, peace, bliss*. Another special mantra was taught to those of us who were ardent spiritual aspirants. I knew my mantras would calm my nerves, as they always did. More than that, I believed they would protect me as our jetliner hurtled through the skies toward a great unknown.

We were on our way to a place I'd been dreaming of visiting for a long while. Shortly after I'd arrived at the Center, Walt and Magaña had announced they were searching for a retreat location in the tropics. They envisioned a place where they could, a few times a year, take small groups of students on respites to dive into the yoga and meditation practices and focus on their health, free of the usual torrent of daily obligations. They explored sites throughout South and Central America, including in Belize, Costa Rica, Guatemala, and Colombia, before purchasing oceanfront property in Magaña's native land. The setting in El Salvador, they'd told us, had everything they'd envisioned and more, including access to the ocean and to lush jungle hiking trails. The property was in the center of three significant volcanoes, an energetically potent location conducive to our spiritual purpose. The country had some known archeological sites, and also held the tantalizing prospect of many ancient treasures that were as yet unearthed. Best of all, it had, as Magaña said, "people with big, beautiful hearts." At the time, of course, no one had any idea that this idyllic country would soon be roiled by a bloody civil war. To the contrary, El Salvador was an up-and-coming travel destination.

From the instant the announcement was made that the retreat plan was becoming a reality, rumors flew around the yoga center and the excitement was contagious. My own heart leapt with joy. But then my hope was threatened by self-doubt. *Why would he pick me?* I thought. *I'm still a new student. So many others are far more advanced and worthy.*

But a small seed was germinating. Although I only had the vaguest idea of where El Salvador was (everything south of Mexico was, at that point, only a vague notion to me), a certainty arose in me that I must and would go there. I would do everything in my power to make it happen. Night after night, I would lie in bed and try to focus every fiber of my being on the idea, and I prayed hard to God to help me make it happen. I felt He was listening. *Salvador*, after all, means "savior" in Spanish.

One by one, during the following year, I bade farewell to the yoga students who were invited to the El Salvador property to work on the building of the retreat. Each one would return after a month or two to the San Francisco Center appearing tan, healthy, and energized, with exotic tales of sleeping in hammocks in the jungle and helping native workers clear the land of thick brush and undergrowth over the entire property, from the jungle to the sand's edge. It became clear that the work was physically demanding, but the reward was a fantastic sojourn filled with camaraderie—and enviable guru stories.

I could not imagine being so close to Gurudev on a daily basis and working side by side with him. At the end of each day, the returning students said, Walt would take them all out for a meal and a Pilsener, the local beer that was a great favorite. I listened in silent awe to their anecdotes and tried to imagine myself in a lifestyle that included such close proximity to my teacher.

Now the moment was here. I was actually on my way, and despite being airborne, I wanted to feel grounded. I repeated my mantras, but my mind wandered like a hobo. I hopped on train after train of memory. Even the mantras themselves got me reminiscing.

Like many spiritual teachers, Walt espoused the power of mantras. These short combinations of sacred words were meant to be repeated with the tongue of the mind—repeated until the speaker connected with the meaning of each word and finally *became* the embodiment of what each word represented.

"Mantras wear a groove in the brain, in the cells," he told us. "They can reverse a negative thought pattern that's been with you your entire life. It's not possible to feel negative when your mind is embracing words like *peace, harmony,* and *well-being.* It's not possible to feel faithless or cynical when you're reciting *joy, peace, bliss.* By choosing the mantra, you choose the direction you want your mind to go."

When I first heard the mantras Walt recommended, a part of me wondered why they didn't sound more esoteric. I'd heard of mantras, as many had, not long after the Beatles had journeyed to India in the 1960s. But weren't they supposed to be comprised of mysterious Sanskrit words? And weren't they supposed to be secrets—transmitted privately, with the receiver forbidden to reveal them?

But the ever-practical and down-to-earth Walt knew that words in any language, English included, could pack a potent—even a divine—punch. (Using the same rationale, he eschewed the practice of using, or conferring on his followers, spiritual names other than their birth names. "What's wrong with your name?" he would ask. "Make *it* a spiritual name.")

Walt would also tell us that practicing a mantra was preparation for fielding life's curveballs. You want to develop in the mind a habit of mantra so that finally the mantra repeats itself. "When you find yourself in a difficulty," he assured us, "you'll see how your mind automatically repeats the mantra and it becomes a protection on many planes."

If I had any doubt about the viability of Walt's workaday words, it was eradicated one rainy night as I was driving my old Austin-Healy Sprite across the Golden Gate Bridge to visit a friend in Sausalito. Just as I was about to reach the end of the bridge, my car hydroplaned on the slick road and I was struck from behind by another vehicle. The impact wasn't great, but it was enough to send me careening across three lanes of traffic, unable to regain control of the wheel. I didn't think—there was no time for anything so complicated—but I spontaneously began shouting my mantra. Somehow my car, seemingly with a mind of its own, and with cars whizzing around me, straightened itself out, eased over to the far right lane, and guided itself down an exit ramp where it came to a stop on the shoulder.

Of course, had Walt been another kind of spiritual teacher, I might never have been out and about in the world availing myself, literally, of spiritual road tests. Many students who study with the great masters lead a cloistered existence while they do so. Secluding themselves in monasteries or ashrams, they become "renunciates," cutting themselves off indefinitely from friends, family, income-earning vocations, and all material concerns. As I would soon discover, this type of seclusion can yield many benefits. But while we were at the San Francisco center, Walt wanted us out in the world, bringing all we learned to every area of our lives. "We don't grow hothouse yogis here," he'd say. "Orchids wilt in the streets of the city. It's far more difficult to maintain your spiritual practices in the midst of the world. But in this lifetime, your work is in the world. You will be stronger for it." Walt had no problem with merging material and spiritual success. His golden rule: "Wherever you go in life, it should be a better place because you were there."

It was true that for the past two years I'd spent a great deal of time at the Center working, working out, learning, and socializing with others in the Baptistes' diverse circle. I also devoted time to playing my flute with Magaña's belly dance troupe of thirty dancers and musicians. Nevertheless, I made my rent in a series of small but cozy apartments by supplementing my waitressing income with side jobs offered to me by yogi friends, ranging from construction sander to bookkeeper. I also found time to flirt and date with the usual enthusiasm—and fickleness—of the average twentysomething.

Along with all this, thanks to Walt, who gave me the unheard-of time off, I formally studied what since childhood I thought was my true calling: acting. (The childhood nickname bestowed upon me by my parents was Sarah Bernhardt, and in my heart of hearts I dreamed of becoming another Elizabeth Taylor.) In this profession, I felt, I could put my lifelong sensitivities to other people's emotions to use. But I knew I needed to work on the complexities of the craft, and had begun taking classes at the American Conservatory Theater with an instructor who turned out to be Helen Hayes's son.

I did have the sense, though, throughout all of this, that something somehow was guiding me, looking out for me, and safeguarding me not only from external dangers, like potential car crashes, but from myself—or at least from the parts of myself that were still naïve and immature. At one point, for example, I'd agreed with an aspiring photographer that it might be a good idea to further my acting career by breaking into modeling. A session posing for a few nude photos in exchange for a professional head shot photo shoot could only further my aspirations, right? But the day before the shoot was scheduled, Walt called me out of the blue with a request that I teach his two yoga classes the following morning and evening while he took a trip out of town. Honored beyond belief that I'd been selected to instruct in Walt's stead (and this while I was still a novice), I readily agreed, though it meant canceling with my photographer friend. The cosmic implication of all this was more than clear to me, and as headstrong as I could be, I never for a moment considered rescheduling. The message seemed obvious to me. Once again, I was being divinely protected.

In many ways, I was just like any young person far from hometown and family. I was giddy with newfound freedom, determined to make it on my own (I'd seen my parents as they traveled to nearby venues with the Cleveland Orchestra, but refused to go home for a visit, lest I feel too much like the girl I'd left behind). I was also pretty much incapable of thinking more than a few months into the future. But at the same time, I was evolving on a deeper level. I began to think about unfolding events less as random happenings than as forums for lessons to be learned. When something significant occurred in my life, I would also wonder about the karma from past lifetimes that contributed to what I was experiencing in the present. By no means did I have all the answers, but I certainly had better questions than ever.

I have to admit that I didn't always appreciate, in the moment, the continual cosmic nudges that elbowed me back onto a path that was often rigorous and difficult. I sometimes felt sorry for myself. In those early years of yoga I would move from states of high exaltation and spiritual bliss, in which I was inspired to give my life to grace, to all but forgetting what I was about and wallowing in self-pity at the unfairness of my burdensome life. I'd also conveniently forget that I was doing this thing out of my own free will. I'd flip from having profound insights back into my mundane habitual mental patterns. Poor me.

But Walt was understanding. "Everyone does that," he said. "The challenge is to remember to remember. When you get too far afield, you forget how to pull yourself out. That's why daily practice is so important."

And practice I did, supplementing yoga classes with hours of additional *asanas* and meditation, sometimes at home, and sometimes on my afternoon breaks at nearby Baker Beach. The result was an ever-deeper hunger for an understanding of life's purpose, and for a firsthand realization of God. Yes, I knew these were lofty aspirations. But I felt driven to do whatever it took to get there. I wanted to elevate my consciousness, and I was determined not to be what Walt referred to as a "trained flea."

"You train circus fleas by putting them in a box," he'd explained. "You keep a lid on the box and the fleas can only jump so high. But when you take the lid off the box, they still only jump so high. You are like that in your self-imposed limitations. You are spanked and conditioned by life in so many ways until you behave according to society's expectations. Your beliefs about yourself and life's possibilities are so limited. But once you take up the yoga practices, you are given the means to jump out of the box and really express your true potential. You then live five lifetimes in one, and your true potential begins to express itself in a natural way."

Sometimes I reminded myself that I was still young, and that there was plenty of time to jump higher. But I was impatient. Once, I asked Norman when Walt had gained his insights, and Norman startled me by telling me that Walt had not finished high school, but was brilliantly versed in the classics, with instant recall of philosophical literature. Even without formal training, he had begun teaching when he was seventeen years old.

"Walt called it *sharing*," Norman said. "His father gave him two rooms in the house so he could give metaphysical talks to groups of people." Norman explained that Walt had been born into a family with an interest in spirituality (as the Law of Reincarnation would have it). His uncle, Joseph Baptiste, had been instrumental in bringing Paramahansa Yogananda, whose *Autobiography of a Yogi* had influenced me and countless other seekers, to America in the 1920s.

"Who came to hear a seventeen-year-old teach?" I asked.

"Lots of people. Most of Walt's students were much older than he was, but only if you just count the years in this lifetime."

"You mean Walt had been on earth more times than they had?"

"Let's just say he's an old soul," said Norman. "He's been many places, on many levels of existence. He'll tell you himself that he's here with a 'commission' to help others understand their true nature, to bring out their inner light, and to help them understand what this life really is."

Hearing about Walt's prodigious accomplishments filled me with awe, but also with some degree of insecurity. He was an old soul, so I must be a rookie. But Norman assured me, "Walt only works with people whose souls are already shining through their material bodies."

It was true that Walt, as a true pioneer of the mind-body-spirit outlook that swept the country once the Love Generation came of age, could have become a superstar marketer of spirituality. He never went down that path. Since he and Magaña had opened their first yoga center in the "Dark Ages'" of 1955, it seemed that the people who found him were the ones by whom he'd wanted to be found. And I was one: a finder.

Unlike Walt, when *I* was seventeen I had been consumed with thoughts of boys, clothes, and ways to sneak cigarettes. But maybe I had just briefly detoured off a preordained path. In the course of two years at the Center, I became certain it was that path that led to California. And now it was leading to El Salvador.

When Gurudev *finally* invited me to accompany him to the retreat, I jumped—right out of my box—at the opportunity. I didn't know how long I'd stay, but I assumed it would be a few months, and that was long enough for me to give up my apartment and pack up my few boxes of treasures and store them with a friend. I briefly wondered what those possessions would mean to me when I returned, for somehow I sensed I would be quite different than when my journey began.

And so on this autumn night, as my airplane sped toward the awaiting jungle, I deemed myself ready. I tried again to focus on my prayer beads, but with only modest success. Once I was ready to move on from memories, visions of my destination danced before me, fanning the embers of my inner fire to know more and more—and still more. I imagined El Salvador would be, for me, a period of growth, maturation, and self-mastery, but also a chance for a great adventure. I would not be disappointed on any count. It was in this tiny Central American country, far from civilization, that I would receive training and initiation into inner spiritual practices that would be nearly impossible for me to experience in the midst of a worldly life. I would need, for a time, to give up the world as I knew it to return to it transformed.

PART II

God-Mad in El Salvador

CHAPTER 9

STARGAZING

"All other paths must one day wind up at the feet of practice."
—WALT BAPTISTE

*O*ur plane touched down at El Salvador's international airport at 6:05 in the morning, and I stepped out into a kaleidoscope of sensation, briefly recalling the scene in *The Wizard of Oz* where Dorothy's world shifts from black and white to vivid Technicolor. In the distance I saw a huge volcano, framed by patches of gardenias, hibiscus, and bougainvillea trees.

As we walked across the tarmac into the airport, the feel in the air, saturated with floral scents and sultry tropical humidity, was unlike anything I'd encountered. It was spring in El Salvador, the coolest time of the year. The rainy season had just ended and it would be several months before the sweet stickiness would build to a steamy crescendo; even so, and even at this early hour, the atmosphere was moist and thick. I imagined I might be able to reach out and wring a chunk of space with my hands until droplets fell to the ground.

But beyond what I was taking in with my five senses, something more was going on. It was as if I had not just swapped locales, but also dimensions. In a matter of moments, I had been catapulted into a state of consciousness in which I felt more present and more connected to life than I had ever been.

Once inside the antiquated airport, I studied my fellow Salvadoran travelers as we waited for our luggage. Most were diminutive compared to my five-foot-seven stature. Many in the crowd sported spike heels and fashionable jeans with designer logos. Despite the early morning hour and general lack of sleep among the passengers, there was a palpable energy as they chattered with one another, obviously happy to be home.

In 1976, exciting things were happening in this tiny country, which had yet to find itself in the turmoil that would eventually catapult it into international view. At this moment, El Salvador was on the verge of moving squarely into the international tourist market and was expectantly preparing itself to handle the throngs of travelers soon to arrive. Global hotel chains were opening—deluxe accommodations at bargain prices to entice American vacationers. A major international airport, replacing this more antiquated one, was soon to open near the coast.

After a long wait our bags arrived, and the customs officer gave us a perfunctory once-over before waving us through. When we walked out the door into the fresh tropical morning, I noticed a few soldiers with large guns standing sentry. But since no one seemed to pay the slightest bit of attention to them, I shifted my focus to the happy crowd of Salvadorans greeting arriving friends and family with a fiesta welcome.

Following Walt's lead, Sandra, Marina, and I piled into a large and dusty old taxi while the driver tied our excess luggage to the roof. Walt sat in front, and we three huddled in the back. The trip took about an hour and a half. For the first hour, we

coasted along a modern two-lane highway that curved precariously around a mountainside as it wound its way down to the
ocean. Several times, our driver quickly made the sign of the
cross before veering around blind curves. Fortunately, I was too
absorbed in the world outside the window to pay much attention to his concerns.

El Salvador was waking up. Alongside the road, women were
selling coffee, fresh coconuts, and tortillas in makeshift stalls,
hoping to make a few *colones* from locals walking to the fields
to begin a day's labor. In front of roughly built shacks, several
small, round-bellied children ran laughing circles around clus-
ters of pigs and chickens. I opened my dusty window to get
a clearer view of the countryside and a fresh blast of intense
color and scent rushed in. Nature's raw life force was overpowering. It was as if we had stepped back into another time,
another century, when earth still overshadowed man instead of
the other way around.

At one point, I spotted a curious homemade sign that read
"PYRAMID," with an arrow pointing to a mound of earth
in an empty field. Walt explained that it was in this part of the
world that the ancient Mayan civilization reached its zenith. A
few pyramids had since been unearthed and opened to the public, but hundreds remained hidden. As we drove along I envisioned another time, its artifacts now buried under a thin layer
of earth, where a people lived out their lifetimes with an acute
understanding of the essence of life's meaning. I could only
guess at the treasures that lay covered beneath the surface.

After about an hour, we abruptly took a turnoff onto a dirt
road so bumpy that the taxi only managed to rattle along at
four miles an hour. The car stirred up a huge cloud of dust, and,
with my window still open, I could taste the dry earth in my

mouth. The unpaved road wound past a series of cotton fields and then cut a swath between two ominous-looking jungle marshes before veering off onto a route parallel to the sparkling ocean. It took thirty minutes to go the two-mile distance, but our agitated stomachs seemed a small price to pay once we were delivered to our destination.

The front gates of the retreat, decorated on either side with fuchsia-colored bougainvillea bushes, were opened by a friendly looking Salvadoran who Walt proudly introduced as the retreat *guardián*, Fernando. Standing beside Fernando was his wife, Anna, and their two little girls, Julissa and Sylvia. They were all genuinely happy that Señor Baptiste had returned. Walt greeted each one warmly and reached down to place a colorfully wrapped candy in each child's small hand. He was rewarded with giggles and sparkling eyes.

As introductions were being made all around, my old friend Matthew bounded out from one of the buildings. I'd been longing to see Matthew since he'd taken leave from his job as head chef at the Hungry Mouth to serve as manager of the retreat. He looked tan and healthy and was teeming with energy, although I imagined he had been on overdrive for days as he readied everything for the guru's return.

"Welcome back, Walt," Matthew grinned, almost shyly.

Walt beamed back at him. "You look terrific, Matthew. Thank you for taking such great good care of everything and everyone."

Matthew was practically bursting with happiness as he accepted Walt's compliment. Then he turned to us with a huge smile. "Welcome to El Salvador." Part of me wanted nothing more than to run up to Matthew and throw my arms around him, but I managed to curb my impulse, remembering that Walt discouraged physical displays of affection between students, preferring subtler heart-energy connection instead.

Matthew ushered us to our rooms to drop off our bags, then steered us to the kitchen where he quickly whipped up a breakfast of eggs, tortillas, and local red beans. I ate ravenously, partly because of the long journey and partly because the eggs were more delicious than any I'd ever had. The eggs were from our very own chickens, I was told. And the creamy milk we drank was from our very own goats.

After breakfast, Walt had us meet him at the beach for a quick dip in the ocean. He explained that there were strong currents offshore and warned us to take care. In the coming year, I would find out just how serious this warning was to be taken, but that day I was mostly mesmerized by the incredible roar of the waves, which seemed to permeate my every cell. Walt told us he'd meet us that night, and every evening, on the beach for a sunset meditation. But right then, he wanted to give us the grand tour of the property.

When we'd dried off, Walt proudly showed us around the entire retreat, much of which was still a work in progress. The retreat was comprised of four one-acre lots. One lot was beachfront property, and on it was a small house for the *guardián*, as well as Walt and Magaña's house. The Baptistes' house, with an image of the sun etched into its stucco facade, was actually built on the second story above a large, overhanging arch. When you walked through the arch, you entered a courtyard, sheltered from the sun by a canopy of almond trees. Brilliantly colored bougainvilleas and exotic tropical plants surrounded a large wooden aviary. The courtyard was filled with a variety of plants and miniature water features. Carefully placed among the plantings were several small sculptures created by Walt, meant to portray apparitions of celestial beings he'd encountered in his meditations.

The courtyard was surrounded by a horseshoe-shaped brick structure that would house students in single and double rooms. On the ground floor of the left side of the horseshoe was a Japanese-style meditation room with *shoji* screens, large paper lanterns, hanging blue and pink wall tapestries, bamboo practice mats, and an altar bedecked with pictures of great Indian yoga masters like Sri Ramakrishna, Kirpal Singh, and Swami Sivananda, the last of whom was influential in bringing the teachings of the Hindu scriptures to the West. On the ground level of the right-hand side of the horseshoe was the pristine kitchen, complete with a gleaming stainless steel double sink, a large refrigerator-freezer, and a four-burner portable electric stovetop. The only modern convenience that was lacking, I learned, was hot water—but boiling water to wash dishes seemed like a fittingly exotic activity. The adjacent dining salon had ten good-sized tables and many tall wooden chairs that would, I was soon to learn, play a central role in my daily life. At the far end of the room, neatly stacked on shelves, was an array of books left behind by previous visitors and a regulation Ping-Pong table.

The remaining three acres were just across the road, bordered at the back by a high brick wall separating the property from the *estero*, a muddy jungle swamp that ran the property's length. Here, in the back of the property, was a large chicken coop built up against the wall. Next to it was the goat pen. Roadside, a gate opened onto a crystal clear pool surrounded by a few well-appointed cabana suites and a simple but well-equipped free-weight gym with a warped hardwood floor that had been damaged during the previous rainy season.

"We're learning about the intensity of the forces of nature here as we go," Walt noted soberly. "Magaña planned to have the gym double as a dance studio. Now, we'll have to pull the floor up and leave it concrete." An expensive lesson here in the jungle.

Walt had detailed plans to add more features to this part of the property, so now, local workers were adding additional guest quarters to this side of the compound. When we would approach a building site, I would look at it from the outside. Walt would invariably enter the doorway or whatever entry was available and firmly plant himself in the middle. "Don't just look from the outside," he admonished, "come inside of it and be in the center of it. Be a part of it. Feel it." He introduced us to each of the workmen, and as we took in our new surroundings, he made the time to personally connect with each man, asking about his family or listening thoughtfully to their construction suggestions. At the time, Walt's Spanish was still limited, but he made each one of them feel important, forging a heart communication that transcended language.

In the course of the morning I was introduced to the animals that shared this bit of land with us. Besides the boisterous chickens and rambunctious goats, there were cats, dogs, and birds. The retreat's lush aviary, directly outside my room, was inhabited by a rainbow of raucous parrots, most of them living in separate cages. Despite their bravado, they were lorded over by a tiny owl, Angel, who was wise enough to form a special bond with Magaña and displayed as much by riding around on her shoulder at every opportunity. The owl had been brought to Magaña as an orphaned fledgling and she hand-fed it with an eyedropper until it was old enough to eat. Walt's giant macaw, Pancha, held court in a large suite next to the parrots.

Our acreage was also home to a number of local cats that had gravitated to it over the course of the past year. Two dogs, large, caramel-colored shepherd mixes that Walt named Amigo and Maya, gifted to Gurudev by a neighbor, had become his special companions—and they looked well fed enough to prove it.

Our first few days were filled with outings. Walt familiarized Sandra, Marina, and me with the lay of the land. Meanwhile, we novices acclimated to the tempo of El Salvador, a languid pace rooted wholly in each unfolding moment. We watched women in simple button-down-the-back dresses grinding fresh corn for tortillas that they would stuff with meat and cook up as *pupusas*. We saw straw-hatted men walking oxen, keeping the beasts in line with gently flicking switches. Everyone seemed somehow dreamy and graceful, and as I took it all in, I felt myself slowing and savoring each sight. My very vision seemed to sharpen, as if I'd been given a new pair of glasses and realized that I hadn't actually been seeing properly for a long time.

We ambled up and down the beach, where many native Salvadorans had their own vacation houses—most unoccupied at this time of year. We explored San Salvador, the capital city, and visited La Libertad, a coastal resort town only eight miles from the retreat. La Libertad was a weekend vacation spot for city dwellers and for itinerant surfers in search of the perfect wave. The town had a sleepy ambience, but Walt told us that it changed character dramatically to a fun-filled holiday spot on Saturdays and Sundays, its ranks swelling well beyond its official population of ten thousand. We sampled the center of town at a quiet time, strolling down narrow streets lined with faded pastel structures, remnants of Spanish influence. As in most Spanish colonies, La Libertad was built around a town square. On one side was the Catholic church. The modern, open-air structure was the square's focal point. Its elegant contemporary design and its cleanliness stood in stark contrast to the dusty and anti-quated adobe shops surrounding it.

Adjacent to the church was the *mercado*, or town market. Walt had given the market quite a build up, and I was filled with happy anticipation as we approached. Every vegetable and fruit imaginable, I was assured, could be found there during one season or another. El Salvador was known in the region for its variety of fresh produce. Watermelons, mangos, oranges, papaya, Guatemalan apples, tiny bananas, breadfruit, and an array of exotic tropical fruit, as well as almost every leafy green, would be available for pennies.

The *mercado* took up a full city block. On its periphery were vegetable stalls, and at first I assumed this tame open-air scenario was the main market itself. But as Sandra, Marina, and I traipsed behind Walt with empty shopping bags in hand, it was clear there was much more to it. We doggedly followed Gurudev through a small doorway into the central part of the *mercado*, a covered, dark, cave-like interior filled with hundreds of vendors hawking their wares.

The produce at the *mercado*, I immediately saw, lived up to its reputation. The rich volcanic soil clearly had a powerful effect on the life force of the food: the richness of its colors, and the intensity of its scents and tastes were startling. It was as though every fruit I'd ever eaten was a pale imitation of the genuine Eden-like article I found here. But, despite Walt's quaint description of the convivial atmosphere we would find at this place, the rest of the scene struck me as nightmarish.

It was already late morning when we arrived, and the heat was stifling. There was little circulation and the stench of food and flesh was overpowering. For a moment, I thought I would be sick. Raw sides of beef and pork and assorted entrails hung from hooks amidst huge bags of rice, beans, and corn. A man was swatting flies away from his fresh farmer's cheese with little success. A wizened, toothless woman reached out to grab my sleeve, speaking insistently to me in rapid-fire Spanish. It seemed as if everyone was watching me, shouting, and competing with one another for my attention.

Dizzy and confused, I looked around and realized my companions were already far ahead. Praying for strength, I shakily forged forward, thankful that I would never have to come here alone. In fact, if I never had to come here again, I would be forever grateful. I kept my eye on Walt, who seemed to be heading toward an exit, but at the last minute turned to one of the women selling tomatoes. I breathlessly caught up to him. Trying to seem as if I were on top of things, I quickly pointed out that the tomatoes he was about to buy from her were not nearly as beautiful as ones in the stall next to it.

He turned to me and calmly replied, "This woman needs the money more."

On the way out, Walt explained that the women vendors at the *mercado* sat in their stalls from sunrise to sunset. Many of them had begun their day by carrying their goods on a crowded, hour-long bus trip from the Grand Mercado in San Salvador.

"They come even on the hottest days," Walt said. "They come when it's excruciating. But the money they earn buys maize and beans for their families' dinner."

In the months and years to come, I would have ample opportunity to revise my sense of the *mercado*. It never changed, but I did—and that made all the difference in what I saw and what I felt there. But for now, I was just grateful to be able to regain my bearings and my breath.

A few blocks from the square was the ocean. Its proximity was the reason for La Libertad's founding, as the town was formerly the major port for the country. The town's pier still welcomed scores of fishing boats. In the late afternoon the boats, laden with the day's catch, were hoisted up onto the pier. They were brimming with fish of all varieties and hues, and these gleaming prizes became the focal points of back-and-forth bargaining as the townspeople gathered to buy dinner. Once again, life seemed idyllic. But El Salvador, I was learning, was a land full of contradictions. Mansions could line one side of a street, and dirt-floor lean-tos the other. Despite its wealthy class and its increasing tourism trade, this was still a very poor country overall. Only twenty-five percent of the population had electricity, and the minimum wage for a laborer was equivalent to two dollars a day.

Once we had a sense of our surroundings, Marina, Sandra, and I settled into a daily routine. Matthew left for a brief trip to Guatemala, which was part of the convoluted process for renewing a Salvadoran visa after two consecutive ninety-day stays, and so, except for the hired workers, the three of us were alone with Walt.

Early morning and late afternoon would be spent at the beach body surfing, walking, or sunning. And, of course, there was meditation. Because El Salvador is close to the equator, sunset and sunrise were around six o'clock year-round. These times we would gather for practice and instruction.

But there was also work to be done. Walt assigned us a job varnishing the dozens and dozens of dining room chairs. We worked on this for several hours mid-morning and again in the afternoon, reciting our mantras as we swished our brushes back and forth, back and forth. Like so many other activities at the retreat, chair varnishing became a de facto meditation, another chance to practice being in the present and doing each small thing perfectly.

In the evening, Walt cooked dinner for the four of us and then instructed us in a practice known as stargazing. We would ascend to a space we called the "surf room," a two-story building that was the closest structure to the ocean and right on the beachfront. Three sides of the room had huge open cutouts for windows and looked out onto the crashing waves. There we would put down our meditation towels—always the same piece of material so that our energy would be retained—and settle on the floor. Amigo, a constant tagalong, would stretch out in front of Walt, and Walt would stroke the dog as he led us.

"Look into the sky and search for the brightest star," Walt would say. "Gaze into it. Look right at the very center of the center. When it divides, go through it. Another light will appear. Concentrate on the center of that."

We would each pick out a star and make it the sole focus of our senses. Soon, even the piercing roar of the breakers against the shore would seem to fade away.

"Now, close your eyes and find the star within," Walt would continue.

The first few times I tried this meditation, an afterimage of the star from the sky would register behind my shut eyelids for a few minutes—then blackness. Walt would instruct me to repeat what I'd done and hold on to the afterimage as long as possible. But after a few nights, something in me shifted. Once the outer star faded, an inner star began to glow. I started to gain an inkling of the universe within, which I would come to learn was as expansive as the cosmos.

We would spend at least an hour stargazing each evening. Sometimes, Walt would have us begin by gazing not at a star but at a planet.

"If you gaze at a planet you can receive its energies," he told us. "Be aware of this if you decide to use one as your focus." Venus would bring us love and receptivity; Mars is the warrior planet.

Once, I asked him whether it was wise to gaze at the moon, especially a full moon. There must be a reason, I thought, why so many cultures had myths that revolved around the full moon's dark energies. Walt smiled.

"The moon reflects the light of the sun," he said, "but be cautious. When you gaze into it without being aware, you are open to other energies—good or evil—that are drawing on the full moon for personal power. What you receive from the moon depends on intention and awareness. You need to maintain your psychic boundaries—not open up to anything that comes along."

For the time being, I decided to stick with the more straightforward sun and stars.

After about a week, the four of us were well settled into a rhythm. The days began to melt into one another, and I felt myself beginning to slip even more into a Salvadoran mind-set, becoming increasingly in tune with each moment rather than dwelling on the future. I was aware that we were expecting Matthew to come back from Guatemala with his renewed visa any day now, but I lost track of exactly when that was. I didn't think anything about it when my friend's absence lengthened. Then, one day, Matthew appeared, his usual good cheer subdued.

Later that afternoon, Walt asked me to accompany him down to the beach. I didn't have any idea why he extended this offer, but I was thrilled with the prospect of spending a bit of time in his company, which always held the prospect of a one-on-one teaching. We walked down to the shoreline, but rather than walking along the sand, Gurudev waded into the water as far as his waist. Although we were out in the open, this felt extremely private. As always, the pounding waves thundered, and no one could possibly have overheard us even if they were close by.

"Michele," Walt said, "I have a new job for you."

As accustomed as I'd become to varnishing chairs, I found this tantalizing.

"What is it?"

He told me that Matthew's visa had been denied. In the kind of Central American bureaucratic snafu we'd all become accustomed to, he'd been given a few days to reenter El Salvador and collect his belongings. Then he'd have to go home.

"I'd like you to stay here and manage the retreat after I leave."

I was dumbfounded. This was never in my plans. Helper, yes. Manager, no.

Every insecurity imaginable fought to take over my mind.

"You will not be alone, Michele," Walt assured me. "Any questions you have, you need only to listen inwardly and they will be answered."

I nodded, afraid that any other gesture would give away my self-doubt. It was a trait for which Walt had no patience.

CHAPTER 10

ASANAS

"The purpose of Hatha Yoga is to release tension from the physical body so the mind is free to go on."
—WALT BAPTISTE

*T*he morning was fresh and alive with last-minute activity as Walt made preparations to inspire the construction workers to keep up their pace for the three-to-four-month stretch of time he would be in San Francisco. Marina and Sandra had left days ago, and Walt had remained to turn me from eager visitor and erstwhile chair varnisher to the retreat's surrogate supervisor. My education was a work in progress.

"Come with me, Michele," Gurudev said, motioning me to accompany him as he inspected the work and greeted each workman with a smile and words of gratitude. It was clear that the men not only respected Walt but also genuinely liked him. They had seen how hard he himself worked, and how much he relished laughing and relaxing at the end of a hot day. Walt's sweat and his smiles endeared him to the workers, but it was his profound respect for the land that seemed especially to kindle their affection. It seemed as though he had an ancient intuitive connection to this bit of earth. One of the regulars, Vicente, even called him "Papa."

As we inspected each new building in turn, Walt asked the men what they needed. I made quite a show of scribbling copious notes on a spiral-bound pad of what needed to be done, what materials needed to be ordered. Inwardly, though, I was petrified. Once Walt left later that day, I would be the only English-speaking person for miles around. I'd be in the jungles of El Salvador, struggling to string together a few Spanish phrases as I managed a construction site and twenty men who arrived to work six mornings a week, wearing machetes.

"*Señorita Michele*," Walt announced to each of the workmen, "*es encargada.*"

During the past few weeks, I had seen many of these men around the property. I'd also been assigned the job of purser. Saturdays were paydays, and I would dole out cash to each of the men for their labors during the week. But now, their boss was introducing me as the one in charge, his representative while he was back in America.

When our rounds were finished, I was exhausted and hungry. I picked up fresh tortillas from Anna and asked Fernando if he would kindly cut a coconut for me. It always amazed me that he could calculate the exact slice needed to shave off the top, leaving a perfect circle of white meat exposed. "*Gracias,*" I said, as he politely handed me the homegrown coco.

Over a solitary lunch of thick corn tortillas, a bowl of beans, and coco water, I had a chance to mull over the duties I was assuming. *I have my work cut out for me in paradise*, I thought, reviewing my responsibilities for the next three months until Walt's return: overseeing and paying the construction workers, keeping the property and buildings clean with the help of Anna and Fernando, feeding the animals, and making weekly trips into town for food and supplies. But that was not all. Walt had made it clear that my daily weight workouts, yoga, and meditation practices were not to be ignored. In fact, he had given me an assignment that seemed almost unfathomable.

Two days ago, I had taken a short break from chores in the heat of the afternoon, and decided to go to the pool to cool off. The kidney-shaped, crystal clear pool was the jewel of the retreat center. Set off by a low bamboo fence, it was surrounded by lush tropical flowers and plants that provided a circle of beauty and almost total privacy from the rest of the place. I waded into the shallow end, admiring a concrete elephant whose trunk became a fountain spewing crystalline water. At the other end of the pool, guarding the semicircle of steps leading into the water, were two large concrete frogs, also fountains—*aqua sapos,* as one of Anna's two little girls called them, water frogs. I was deep in reverie when I saw that Walt had entered the pool area, too. He waded in beside me.

"Michele," he said, "I've given you a lot of duties."

"Yes," I agreed. *Maybe he's going to lighten my load,* I thought.

"But there is something else you have to do."

I thought, *Oh, no.* But Walt said aloud, "Yes, yes."

"What is it?" I asked.

"You must master Hatha Yoga."

I did not think I heard correctly. To me, this was like saying, "Play all the music ever written, and do it to perfection."

Hatha Yoga comprises the physical postures of yoga. When you assume any of the myriad yogic poses—say a triangle, or a warrior, or a cat and cow—you are performing Hatha Yoga. But that is only the most superficial definition. To take a pose without mindful attentiveness is not true Hatha Yoga. To take a pose without monitoring the breath is not true Hatha Yoga. To hold a pose with the mind wandering or whining, thinking all the while, "I wish it were over, I wish it were over" (a phase all beginners go through), is not yet mastering the practice of Hatha Yoga. Without the right intention and attitude, you can exercise the body in this rudimentary way by moving it this way and that, and this certainly yields some benefits—you become more supple, for example, and your spine strengthens—but for all the good you are doing your spirit, you might as well be walking on a treadmill.

Hatha Yoga, as Walt meant it, is an integral and inextricable part of Raja Yoga, road to the ultimate reality. Step by step, the Hatha discipline helps us overcome our imbalances and over-rule our lethargy and laziness. It purifies us, prepares us for deep meditative practices, and forges a connection between the material body and the richest, if most intangible, resources of our being.

Of course, to truly master Hatha Yoga would take countless lifetimes. I felt dizzy just hearing Walt's pronouncement. But as I should have known he would, Walt had a very specific plan in mind. He named ten postures, or *asanas*, he said he had selected specifically for me. Each would speed my progress on the spiritual path.

The postures Walt assigned were the bridge, the fish, the wheel, the headstand, the cobra, the full lotus, the full lotus in forward bend, and the seated forward bend with two other variations. With the exception of the headstand and classic lotus pose, all were either backbends or forward bends.

In the bridge, you lie on your back with your knees bent, bringing your feet close to your buttocks, and touch your heels with your hands. You press your feet into the ground and push your pelvis toward the sky.

In the fish, you lie on your back with your legs either straight and together or folded and lift your upper body onto your elbows. Bending your neck backward, you rest the crown of your head on the ground.

The wheel is another backbend. Lying on the back with the knees bent and the feet close to the hips, you place your hands in front of your shoulders and lift your body off the ground into a half circle.

The headstand is one of those postures that looks nearly impossible to attain but is actually something most people can train themselves to do incrementally, as I had. You kneel down, make a triangle of your arms on the floor in front of you, and clasp your hands at the apex of that triangle. You place your head in the cradle of your hands, raise your buttocks, and walk your feet forward, until you can lift your legs toward the ceiling. The trick to staying upright boils down to believing you won't topple.

The cobra is assumed by lying face down on the front of the body and placing your hands on the floor in front of the shoulders. You then straighten the arms and slowly lift the upper body toward the heavens.

The lotus, the classic double-cross-legged "pretzel pose" we think of when we picture meditating Buddha statues, is another *asana* that looks intimidating. And for many of us in the Western world who are not accustomed to squatting and who have tight hip joints, it is truly a challenge. But it too can be achieved through small, repeated measures. One hip is often looser than the other, and if you can coax one foot to rest on the opposite thigh, then you are already in half lotus. In time, practicing over and over again, the hips will open and the other leg will follow suit. My assignment involved not only the basic lotus, but also a variation where once I assumed the full lotus,

I was to bend forward until my forehead touched the ground in front of me, my hands resting in front of the head, one palm covering the other.

The seated forward bend, another hurdle for those who are not yet very flexible, requires sitting with the legs straight in front, feet flexed, raising your arms overhead, and then stretching them forward to hold on to your ankles. Using successive deep breaths, you aim to increase your stretch, letting your head relax toward your knees. Walt also gave me two variations of the full forward bend.

In my two years at the Baptistes' San Francisco Center, I had experienced all of these *asanas* many times. Given the nature of Walt's classes, I was sometimes in the poses for many minutes. So nothing about Walt's specific instructions seemed unattainable. That is, until he revealed the last part.

"I want you to work up to holding each of these poses for one hour at a time."

"An *hour*?"

"Yes, and there is something else that is very important," he added. But I was still stuck on the *hour.*

"*Sixty minutes?*" I repeated, as if breaking it down this way would get Walt to see the error he'd inadvertently made.

"Yes, there are sixty minutes in an hour," Gurudev confirmed with a serious tone. "But you're not listening. That's not the most important thing."

"What's the important thing?" I asked, forcing myself to pay strict attention.

"While you are practicing these poses, hold your focus at your forehead center and use the breath to relax deeply in each pose. These *asanas* will open up your spinal centers. Then, when you have completed the postures, you must use your willpower and your *kriya* breath to bring the energy up your spine and to the higher chakras in the head for spiritual breakthrough. It's crucial that you do this or the tremendous sexual energy that you will awaken will be insatiable."

He repeated this again with great seriousness.

"Remember, you *must* bring the energy *all the way up* to the higher spiritual centers in the head, or you will unleash so much sexual energy that no amount of sex would ever satisfy you. It will take over completely."

On one level, I thought I understood what Walt was referring to. As a yoga student and new teacher I had experienced and heard from many practitioners that taking up yoga had increased their energy levels. For some, it also yielded a quite unexpected side effect: a dramatic upswing in sexual desire. Some people experienced this as a pleasurable perk (as did their spouses, or so I was told), but others were confused by it.

"I can't believe what's happened to my sex life in the six weeks since I started taking these classes," one smiling sixty-seven-year-old woman had happily confided to me as she practically skipped down the steps of the yoga center to her car. Then, there was the other side of the coin: "I don't have time to think about sex every ninety seconds," one busy professional woman complained to me. "I feel like a guy!"

Although a surge of sexual desire does not overtake everyone who embarks on the yogic path, it can and does occur. The reason is a force known as *kundalini*. *Kundalini* is a much misunderstood concept. Many people know that it refers to the coiled up spiritual energy that, according to yogic philosophy, resides at the base of the spine. In a lot of Eastern artwork, you will see representations of this energy embodied as the image of a snake. The misunderstanding lies in what this energy is for, and what it is capable of accomplishing. Yes, it is the source of sexual energy, but also of infinitely more.

All sentient beings draw on *kundalini* for life force the way the lamp on your desk draws on the electrical power grid. Without the grid, there is no light. *Kundalini* is actually the subtlest and yet the most powerful energy known to humankind; it is the strongest force on earth or, in fact, in the universe. What is in our spines is more potent than nuclear energy, more formidable than the atomic bomb.

Kundalini itself is neither "good" nor "bad." As with all forms of energy, everything depends on how we use it. The *kriya* breath that Walt was referring to is a secret practice, part of an oral tradition that is passed down from guru to disciple to awaken the *kundalini* and direct it from the lower chakras to the higher spiritual centers in the head.

"The practice of *kriya* yoga should only be undertaken under the direction of a spiritual teacher who can safely guide you," Norman once told me.

"Why?" I'd asked.

"Because if the energy is misdirected, all sorts of problems can arise."

"Like what?"

"I've heard Walt say that there are people in mental institutions because of misdirected *kundalini*. Awakening the *kundalini* through the *kriya* practices is a tremendous responsibility for both the disciple and the teacher. At the same time, it's said to be the quickest route to enlightenment. If you follow the guide exactly, it can open the inner door to spiritual reality."

As I delved into the subject further, I learned that sexual energy and orgasm is *kundalini* energy directed outward into the physical plane. But for the spiritual devotee, this energy can be conserved and directed inward and upward in meditation for the high goal of enlightenment. That is why many monks and swamis practice celibacy: so this precious energy can be used for spiritual breakthrough.

When we awaken a great quantity of *kundalini,* as happens in the kind of intense yogic practice Walt was prescribing for me, we have to be careful not to let this great unleashed force remain in the lower chakras, where it can overstimulate the purely physical appetites. Walt's warning was meant to remind me to take the energies I was about to release and channel them upwards through the chakra system to awaken the higher chakras.

I knew from my years of study that each pose Walt assigned was meant to open up one or more of the seven main chakras— wheels of energy located in the area of the spine and brain that are akin to major power stations along the electrical grid. In addition to opening up the three lower chakras, which are located at the base of the spine, at the level of the genitalia, and at the solar plexus, the *asanas* would open the heart chakra, seat of love and compassion, and the throat chakra, seat of authenticity and truthful speech. At the very highest levels, they would open the brow or "third eye" chakra, the seat of intuition and the opening to divine guidance, as well as the "crown" chakra, the secret opening at the top of the head that allows our energy to radiate upward and merge with the energies of the world beyond us. My practice was designed for nothing less than to help me attain the highest goal of the yogi: spiritual realization.

The morning after Walt gave me my *asanas* assignment, I arose especially early and decided to begin. I fixed my mind on my goal, the reason I was here. *I will do whatever it takes. The guru wouldn't be giving me this practice unless I was ready for it. I can do it, and I will do it.*

I knew I would have to devote much time and energy to these poses after he left, and I saw my upcoming time alone as a God-given opportunity to progress toward knowledge of the divine, to at least gain a glimmer of the spiritual brass ring. My personal training with Gurudev here in El Salvador had already caused major shifts in my health, mental attitude, and perceptions. I felt eager to speed things along, and was determined to follow my teacher's direction to the letter.

But, alone in the meditation room, I struggled. I held each of the postures for a number of minutes, managing to remain in many of them longer than I ever had in the past. But it was hard to bring my energy up. I felt, as Walt had warned me I might, plagued by sexual thoughts. I felt a surge of energy pulsating in my genitals, as if I were on the verge of a climax. I experienced what felt like a reckless and indiscriminate desire. I became distraught and began to berate myself. Why was it so hard to conquer the impulses of my body and my emotions? Lust, hunger, laziness, fear, anger. I felt like a poster child for the seven deadly sins.

But after a while, I calmed myself. I was even able to smile at myself. Evidently, I didn't get all the energy up. Okay, fine. To do this, concepts I had held for a very long time would have to be broken down. In my afternoon session, things went better. I was able to reabsorb some of the sexual current and redirect it. In time, I felt I would be able to do a better job of this, but I knew I would have to be patient. I would have to override my ego, my false concepts of the self, and I would have to let my real Self shine through. It's only by doing this that I could get my body under the clear direction of the mind. Advanced yogis have conquered their bodies utterly. That is why you hear stories—true stories—of Himalayan masters who can slow their hearts and respiration rates to a near standstill, or raise or lower their body temperatures at will.

That night, at dinner, Walt gently reprimanded me. Not surprisingly, he seemed to be aware of my emotional roller coaster ride earlier in the day. While we were eating, he looked over at me and said. "Joy, Michele. You need to know joy inside regardless of how materiality is going."

"I'll try," I said.

"You're not there yet, but you will be," he said. "While you are here, you will be learning about the nature of your mind."

I felt optimistic at that moment, but with Walt about to actually leave, I hoped I could quell my fresh anxieties. I didn't want mental gymnastics to get the better of me. After lunch, I rested awhile and then went back outside. Ducking under a low coconut branch, I opened a bamboo gate and saw Walt, in his bathing suit and handwoven Guatemalan vest, crouching down and carefully examining a small stick poking out of the ground. It was a plumeria branch that he had brought to El Salvador, hoping it would take root in the pool garden and bloom into a fragrantly blossomed frangipani tree. Secretly, I doubted it would make it here. The branch looked to me like a dead stick and nothing more.

He turned and called to me. "Michele, this plumeria isn't being watered properly. I specifically asked Fernando to water it twice a day, but it's very dry. Please see that every plant gets watered properly. It's critical in this climate." His tone was stern and I found myself practically standing at attention. He stood up and walked to two nearby bamboos towering above the other plants. "And these bamboos," he added, "they must also be watered twice a day, and for a good length of time. They need plenty of water, and in the dry season a light spray just isn't enough. I asked Fernando to let the hose run on each one for a few minutes, but keep an eye on them. You can quietly supplement the watering yourself."

Many months would go by before I came to understand that much of what Walt was teaching me about caring for the retreat were metaphors or coded messages for deeper teachings and practices. During these early days, he was creating the language that would later be used to guide me in my spiritual journey.

We walked toward the pool together and he motioned for me to sit beside him on the steps. Together we sat immersed, waist-deep in the water. Overwhelmed with the events of the day and the proximity of my teacher, combined with his near departure, I somehow remembered to silently repeat the mantra. My fears, insecurities, and self-doubts subsided.

Walt turned to me, smiling, his luminous eyes swimming with love, and said, "Thank you." It was yet another reminder that there was nowhere to hide. Not even in my thoughts. And because I trusted my guru more deeply than I have ever trusted another living being, I was at peace with everything that already was and that was to come.

We sat silently in meditation for a few blissful minutes until he was called away by Fernando. The taxi had arrived and it was time to pack the car for the trip to the airport.

CHAPTER 11

A COCONUT FOR CHRISTMAS

December 1976

$\mathcal{M}$*y Dearest Michele!*

I think of you and want all to be well, harmonious, and exceedingly beneficial for you.

You are the protectress there of many ideals that are precious to me for the good, truth, and beauty for many who belong there in God's name. Through you, please extend my affection to all there in human form, in the gardens, in the aviary, sky, ocean, etc. totally! And you <u>*know!*</u> *I love you.*

Be dedicated to your inner Practices. Be idealistic and powerfully real and true to the ideals in the meditation room there inside and out—do your health and physical practices daily in a powerful and dynamic manner.

Every day is a crossroads—in which way do thou goest?

Again my love to all—write and tell of all—
Meditate enough that there is communication
between us besides script.

Gratefully and Love,
Walt Baptiste

Christmas morning, my first Christmas in El Salvador and my first as retreat manager, started out just like all my solitary days. There was no sleeping past 6:00 a.m. The parrots simply wouldn't allow it. They trilled and squawked and, in some cases, spoke aloud. One of my feathered alarm clocks warbled, "Pretty bird, pretty bird," with perfect English diction; another hollered like an old fishwife, "*Hector, dame las tortillas!*"—Spanish for "Hector, give me the tortillas!" I had no idea who Hector was, but I sensed, after four weeks of this routine, that he wasn't going to show. It was my job, one of my many jobs, to bring the birds their daily rations of tortillas, corn, fruits, and greens. Each bird, I soon learned, had a distinct personality and unique way of relating to me.

Once, Anna had come up behind me as I was preparing to open one of the cages to hand a piece of tortilla to the large parrot who called out for Hector. "*Pájaro muy bravo,*" she pronounced dramatically. *Very brave bird*, my mind translated as I opened the cage. No sooner did the cage door open but the bird lunged at my wrist and sunk its beak deep into it, hanging on for dear life. The pain was searing and I quickly pulled my hand back with the bird hanging from it. Blood spurting from my wrist, I whipped my hand through the air until the bird let go and dropped to the ground, cackling like the Wicked Witch of the West. Fernando came running and managed, with a very long pole, to get the parrot back in his cage. To this day, I still bear a scar reminding me that the Spanish word *bravo* means "mean," not "brave."

Today, even though it was Christmas, Vicente, the only other regular household employee besides Anna and *guardián* Fernando, arrived early to remove the leaves from the courtyard garden and to sweep and mop the green tile walkways around the compound. He reminded me of Norman, conscientiously sweeping debris from the windy sidewalk of the San Francisco yoga center. And as Norman had done, he brought to my mind an image of a Japanese Zen head monk, whose auspicious duty it is to rake the monastery sand garden at sunrise. Vicente's short, round figure was unmistakable as he diligently performed his tasks. He always wore a broad-brimmed straw hat for protection against the searing sun. And he was always clothed in dusty pants and a worn short-sleeved white shirt that barely buttoned over his large belly.

Vicente had only one arm. His left arm had been bitten off below the elbow by a dog when he was just seven years old. He accepted his fate and lived his life without complaint. He was "married" to Fernando's sister. Formal marriage in El Salvador was next to impossible for the native people because the law insisted that a civil ceremony take place before a church ceremony. The cost of the civil ceremony was fifty dollars, out of the question for most of the *campesinos*.

Gurudev and Vicente had a special relationship of mutual fondness. Vicente worked directly for Walt and was not under the direction of any of the other workers. He was deeply courteous and grateful to be working at the retreat. His devotion and love for Walt was evident, and he told me once that Señor Baptiste was a man of God. *He knows,* I thought. *He's been given an experience.*

After wishing Vicente *Feliz Navidad,* I headed for the gym and began the workout Walt had designed for me. Using five-pound dumbbells, a light body bar, and the other basic equipment, I did a dozen exercises, twenty repetitions apiece. The mindful bending, twisting, and lifting, along with the all-important breath work, got my blood flowing and balanced my energies. Before he left, Walt had said, "Work out every day and things will come together for you in about a month." As usual, he had been prescient. With every passing week I was becoming stronger, not just physically but emotionally and psychically. My initial shyness and uncertainty around the workmen was on the wane. And my level of patience for spiritual practices had grown. That was a very good thing, for along with my long list of managerial duties, these practices occupied hour upon hour of my time.

At nine o'clock each night I practically fell into bed, exhausted from following the strict schedule I'd set for myself. After my morning workout I fed the animals, did my first round of yoga postures, and, typically, had a light breakfast of eggs (if the chickens had cooperated) or a blender drink (if the hens withheld). After breakfast I checked on the workmen's progress, did more yoga, and fixed a light lunch, perhaps a tortilla and a banana or salad and small bowl of beans. Then, I did my *mala* beads and mantra practice and more yoga. After this, I studied Spanish from a workbook, diligently conjugating *-ar* verbs, *-ir* verbs, and *-er* verbs. Then I checked on the progress of the workmen again and fed the animals again. At the end of the day, I sat for sunset meditation, prepared a simple dinner—sometimes fish netted by Fernando in front of the property—and then did more *asana* and *kriya* practice, ending with the stargazing practice Walt had taught me. If the power was on—a big *if* in El Salvador, where a squall or a stiff breeze could knock the electricity out for days at a time—I might look at my Spanish again before turning in, on the theory that the language would permeate my gray matter while I slept. If the power was off, I'd grab a flashlight and ready a jug of bottled water for morning coffee, which would have to be made over the *guardián*'s open fire.

My schedule was sacrosanct. Apart from the one day a week I altered my solitary routine for a supply-gathering trip to La Libertad, you could have set a watch by my crisscrossings of this four-acre universe. Years later, I read *Walden* and was struck by Thoreau's contention that anyone undergoing an extended period of solitude must set a daily schedule for themselves or go mad. It was I who shaped the specifics of my daily agenda, but I sensed even back then that Walt had given me guidelines about what had to be done, for the retreat and for myself, with the purpose of keeping me on track. Alone in the tropics, I would not succumb to beach brain or wallow in the doldrums. In fact, I'd never felt more focused or more organized.

Of the many practices Walt had assigned me, the one I savored and looked forward to from the moment I opened my eyes in the morning was working on holding my yoga poses for extended periods of time. I fit in at least three sessions a day, each one lasting ninety minutes to two hours, and brought a little clock into the yoga room to keep track of my time in each pose. I decided to organize these sessions by working on a small group of poses at a time. Beginning with bridge, headstand, forward bend with variations, and lotus, I first settled into the poses physically and then attempted to get hold of my unruly mind.

The clock was my gauge for the physical aspect of the practice, but the amount of time I was able to hold the physical pose was directly dependent on whether my mind would allow me to do it. Once my body settled into the pose, a fierce competition ensued between my higher mind and my lower mind—between compassionate awareness and a chattering, compromising mind that tried to talk me out of staying with it.

The mental part was the most challenging. At first some of the poses seemed easy, but after ten minutes my mind was screaming so loud I could barely stay present in the situation. I told myself, *Relax, let go, be well.* I would try to stay aware of the situation and not react from a place of pain, suffering, and misery. "Every posture in yoga," Walt taught in a San Francisco class, "brings out a different part of the mind and emotions. When you replace these unconscious habits of thinking with positively charged words, you actually reprogram your subconscious mind."

This tropical retreat setting was a laboratory to experience these truths for myself, and the lessons were loud and clear. Day after day, holding the same pose, I watched similar thought patterns emerge. Fear, self-doubt, insecurity, anger, and frustration all reared their ugly heads. My mind was embroiled in the schemes and compromises of a zillion thoughts encouraging me—no, insisting—that life would be a lot easier if I came out of the posture and got back to it later. It was then that I would hear Walt's voice in my head. "You think if you change positions, life will be simple, that the grass will be greener on the other side of the fence. Instead of building tension, breathe, relax, and let go through the difficulty to the place where all is ideally well. Peace, harmony, well-being, instead of all the yelling and screaming."

As I moved toward the thirty-minute mark, I was able to observe my mind relaxing and to feel a corresponding release in my nervous system as I settled into a new level of tranquility. Toward the end of each session, I heeded Gurudev's directive to bring the energy to the sixth chakra, the third eye chakra, and end in meditation.

Through these intense periods of practice, I came to see that each moment truly is a crossroads, as Walt had written in the very first letter he had sent to me here in El Salvador. It was my choice to buy into the tricks of my mind or to practice staying present and conscious with each passing instant, each passing thought. *Which way does thou goest?* Here, on my own, I would have to continually choose.

Solitude suited me. For most of my life I had surrounded myself with people and endless activities, almost compulsively. I dreaded feeling lonely. Now, the woman who avoided being alone at all cost had completely disappeared, and I reveled in the clarity of mind that was emerging. I began to know what the Bible refers to as the "peace that passeth all understanding." In the weeks since Walt had left, I'd begun to feel I'd taken root in paradise, the never-ending ocean roar an eternal "Om" that tethered me to this place. I felt like I belonged here, and every creature and person around me seemed to accept me as a natural part of the landscape. The dogs, especially Amigo, had become my constant companions, trailing me as they'd shadowed Walt. Up and down the pristine beach, everyone I encountered—the neighbors, their children, the fishermen, and passing townspeople—greeted me as "Señorita Michele." I was a fixture, a sight as familiar as the sparkly sand. I was sun-baked, shoeless, and utterly blissful.

Over the course of the past few weeks, my own perceptions

had altered dramatically. My maiden voyage to the *mercado* in La Libertad with Walt had been a deeply unnerving affair, an event I hoped never to repeat. But a weekly sojourn to the market to fetch food and supplies was one of my responsibilities. The first few times I had left my protected Eden for the raw world of *campesinos* were still unsettling. Now this world, too, was becoming a home to me.

My market days were distinguished by rituals of their own. I was careful to eat a hearty breakfast of tortillas and eggs to ground myself for the onslaught of people and activity. It was important to strike out from the retreat early in the morning, for soon after that the heat would take its toll. I'd walk a mile down the beach toward the small coastal village of Playa de San Diego, where an 8:00 a.m. bus would take me the rest of the way. To get to the village, it was necessary to cross an estuary that ran into the sea. In the rainy season, the water might be so high it could only be crossed by a rowboat—available solely at the whim of its owner. But at this time of year, if my timing was right and the current was not too strong, I took off my clothes, under which I wore a bathing suit, placed my clothes, shoes, money and shopping basket on top of my head, native style, and waded across neck-deep water to the waiting bus.

The first time I set eyes on Playa de San Diego, I was as shocked as I was when I first walked through the *mercado* in La Libertad. A long row of well-tended villas, empty at this time of year, lined the ocean side of the road, but across from them was a long row of dirt-floored cardboard shacks. Pigs and chickens ran loose everywhere, their excrement littering the streets. Naked children with distended bellies rolled in the dirt as their parents gazed on. The air was infused with thick smoke from open cooking fires. I never imagined myself getting used to this village, let alone looking forward to visiting. But already, I was beginning to register the sensations of San Diego through a filter of acceptance and affection. The children's laughter, the women's joking and chatter, the animals' antics, and the aroma of fried *pupusas* combined to make me feel even more alive.

If I had time, I'd take a few minutes before boarding the bus and buy a cold drink at a tiny store run by two elderly sisters. One of them, the one who wore glasses as thick as the Coke bottles in her small generator-run refrigerator, would attempt to fill me in on the week's gossip as I sipped my soda. I barely knew what she was saying, but it was always a happy interlude. I had come to truly relish my six-day stretches of near-silence and, in fact, later noticed that it took me days to recover my calm and clarity when English-speaking visitors came to the retreat. But on town days, bursts of local babble revived me. I once spent the twenty-five-minute bus trip to the port of La Libertad jiggling a newborn baby on my lap as the proud mother told me the story of the birth. I certainly did not catch every word, but I did understand when the boy had been born: *ayer*, yesterday. He was less than twenty-four hours old, and an uncomplaining passenger.

On Christmas morning there would, of course, be no trip to town, and no need to check in on the retreat's construction workers, since everyone had the day off. With some rare free time on my hands, I decided to linger with the birds after I fed them. The parrots, I'd discovered, were music fans and so, straight from the weight room, I went back to my own room to collect my flute. As I walked, Amigo and Maya fell in beside me, expectantly eying their dog food bowls, which I dutifully filled. Amigo ate quickly and started to trail me again within minutes. Maya, who was expecting puppies, lay down for a nap.

hat will we play for *los pájaros* today, Amigo?"

Let out a soft "Boof." I always had the feeling he loved to be consulted on such important matters. And why not? As Walt laughingly pointed out once, the word "dog" is "God" spelled backwards.

The birds had their definite musical preferences. Through trial and error I'd discovered they loved Mozart, were indifferent toward Bach, and went absolutely gaga for *The Sound of Music's* "Do-Re-Mi." This being Christmas, I decided on Mozart's *Adagio Religioso*. This was a piece my father always loved to play, and it served to remind me that for the first time, I would not be in touch with my family on Christmas Day. La Libertad was the closest place I could make a phone call to the States. Once a month, as scheduled, or in an emergency if one arose, I would have to walk a mile down the beach to Playa de San Diego, cross the *estero*, take the bus, go to the phone company—a cramped office near the pier—where I could wait for up to two hours before the call would go through. Cash only. This was my only "immediate" link to Walt, or anyone else.

But I did not feel lonely this Christmas, just as I had not felt lonely since being here. I was, for the first time in my life, developing a relationship with myself rather than with others. But I was far from alone. I leaned heavily on an abiding sense of trust in my teacher, on God, and on the Divine Mother.

The Divine Mother, whom Walt had specifically reminded me to call upon, was becoming increasingly meaningful to me. This feminine aspect of the sacred, the protectress of the universe and the giver of mercy, has been revered in nearly all spiritual traditions in forms ranging from Artemis to the Buddhist Tara to the Virgin Mary. She is Quan Yin, the maternal goddess of compassion who sits on the altars in Chinese temples. In Sanskrit, she is Padma-pâni, "Born of the Lotus," and her cupped hands form the Yoni Mudra, symbolizing the womb as the door for entry to this world through the universal female principle.

Contemplating the Divine Mother, as my guru had instructed me to do, involved no ritual or special practice. She was charged with holding the entire world together, and I was charged with caretaking a very, very tiny piece of it. Had I been working in an office, she would have held a spot near the apex of my organizational chart. I felt she was always with me, tending me as I tended the retreat. I relied on her for guidance and compassion, but I also had often fallen into the habit of calling on her directly when I needed some immediate, practical assistance. If I'd misplaced something, I'd send up a brief plea to the Divine Mother to help me find it. Invariably, it would turn right up.

After my ad hoc concert in the aviary, Amigo and I headed for the chicken coop, where I fed the hens and roosters some *verdolaga* greens and a ration of ground corn.

"*Hola, gallinas. Tenéis algunos huevos hoy?*" Do you have any eggs today?

Spying a half dozen plump, cream-colored prizes, I whooped aloud. Here was a true Christmas present. Before leaving, Walt had reminded me many times to check for eggs each morning. Sometimes there were eggs, sometimes there were not. At first, their presence or absence seemed random. But lately, I'd sensed a pattern. The eggs seemed to materialize when my practices and my duties were going well, when my will was strong, and my mind was clear. The nests remained bare during times when I had been unsure of myself or ego driven, like when Fernando had behaved menacingly during the full moon, drinking to excess and nearly running me over with his bicycle, and I had failed to intervene despite feeling I should. The morning after, no eggs. A few times I'd let Anna talk me out of a promise I'd made to Walt about the apportioning of supplies. Again, no eggs. So today, I was overjoyed with the hens' seeming vote of confidence. I collected my bounty—still warm!—and carefully carried the eggs to the kitchen. But I would not eat them, not yet.

For the past five days I had been fasting on coco water. Every two hours or so, I'd drink a glass of this thin, opaque liquid taken from young, green coconuts. Sweet and vaguely almond-flavored, this beverage alone sustained me in the absence of any solid food.

Walt had introduced me to the astounding benefits of coco water. When he first mentioned it, I thought he was referring to coconut milk, the thick, white liquid made from the meat of coconuts. But coco water was another thing entirely, and more nutritious by far.

"It's the fluid of life," Walt said. "It's full of pure natural sugars, salts, and vitamins. It will give you an incredible energy level."

He also told me that coco water had been used as a plasma substitute during World War II by doctors throughout the South Pacific when they needed to give emergency transfusions to wounded soldiers.

As ever, Walt practiced what he preached. He never failed to drink at least a quart of coco water a day when he was at the retreat. Fortunately, this was one item that was never in short supply. It takes up to a year for coconuts to mature, but the trees bloom up to thirteen times a year and they yield a continual harvest. An average tree would provide us with about sixty coconuts across the four seasons. In addition, I often picked up a dozen on trips into town.

I had become a devotee of fasting since Norman coached me
through my first juice fast in San Francisco, back when I was
quitting smoking. The practice never failed to make me feel
lighter in body and soul. The body expends so much energy
digesting food; when that energy is redirected, repair and res-
toration take place. Now, as always, I was finding that my Spar-
tan regime enhanced my meditation practices. But, all things in
moderation—in the afternoon, I would break my fast. After all,
it was Christmas.

Right then it was time for my *mala* beads practice, then more
Hatha Yoga. After that, I would take up one of my weekly
chores: cleaning and sweeping out the meditation room.
Though Anna did most of the cleaning, this particular task was
mine alone. It was part of my Karma Yoga, my service to the
teachings, and I treated it as yet another sacred practice, sweeping and reciting *peace, harmony, well-being* with the tongue of my
mind.

As I worked I heard another mantra of sorts. The dogs were
not allowed in the meditation room, and Amigo was waiting
patiently outside, sighing at regular intervals to let me know
he was still hopeful of a reprieve. I smiled and, still in holiday
mode, decided to next spend some time engaging in one of his
favorite activities. To be honest, this decision to cheer up Amigo
fell into the realm of enlightened self-interest, for the thing he
liked to do best was to nudge me back and forth while I swung
in a hammock and looked out over the sea.

Looking over the shoreline, alone but for my dear four-
legged friend swinging me back and forth, back and forth, I felt
more content than I ever had. Far in the distance, I could see
the outline of La Libertad and a few fishing boats heading back
to the pier, but this world seemed a million light years from

mine. I had everything I needed, everything I could have ever wanted. Soon, soon, when the sun went down, I would break my fast with the succulent meat of a ripe coconut. I would sit in the warm sand with Amigo wrapped around my feet, I would count my blessings, and I would gaze at a star, a Christmas star.

My mind drifted to Walt's teachings of the three wise men who followed the star to find the Christ, "the light of the world." The Christmas star that the Magi followed represents the star that appears inside in meditation. The spiritual devotee who focuses on the inner star will come to Light within. This, then, was the essence of the stargazing practice he had left me with.

The hammock slowed down and stopped, pulling me back to the present. Amigo had decided it was time for his Christmas dinner and was letting me know it in no uncertain terms. As the sun began its descent toward the edge of the sea, the birds started up an excited conversation, anticipating their afternoon feast. "*Hec-tor,*" screamed the *muy bravo* bird. The others squawked in response.

I leapt out of the hammock, fed everyone their meals, and headed to the beach with my precious Christmas coconut, a satisfied Amigo proudly marching by my side. I sat for sunset meditation as usual, fingering the holy prayer beads my guru had given me and beginning the repetition of my mantra. At first, my concentration failed. I noticed that the holiday was causing my mind to wander ahead. I thought of the new year and what it would bring. But I pulled myself back from the unknown future. *Peace, harmony, well-being.* I made each word a perfect pearl, until on the wings of their rhythm my mind rested in the perfect present.

CHAPTER 12

REUNION

*"Those whose consciousness is unified abandon all
attachment to the results of action and attain supreme
peace. But those whose desires are fragmented, who are
selfishly attached to the results of their work, are bound
in everything they do."*

—THE *BHAGAVAD-GITA*

*B*ack home, as the first months of 1977 unfolded, Jimmy
Carter was sworn in as the thirty-ninth president of the United
States. *Roots* became a blockbuster miniseries. The Eagles's *Hotel
California* ruled the pop charts, and everyone danced to Donna
Summer. In Cupertino, California, a new company, Apple
Computer, Inc., was busy being born. John Travolta was making *Saturday Night Fever*, and George Lucas was getting ready to
release the first *Star Wars*. As for me, I might as well have been
in a galaxy far, far away. I was twenty-eight years old with no
love life, no traditional job, no money to speak of. I was oblivi-
ous to the American Dream. I did not crave a house, a car, a
high-powered career. I continued to dream only of one thing:
reaching, one day, the pinnacle of spiritual insight.

The more weeks that passed, and the more that silence and
solitude became my prevalent state, the more I felt myself

blossoming. Except for the increasing humidity signaling the approaching rainy season, living in paradise suited me, and I spent each day immersed in the fragrant smells and brilliant colors of the tropics, with the ever-present sound of the ocean's distant roar in the background enveloping every corner of my being. I felt buoyantly healthy and light, and although I rarely glanced in a mirror, I suspect I never looked better. No matter that there was no boyfriend to appreciate my allure. With my *kundalini* redirected, I didn't think much about sex anymore. Walt had never dictated rules related to his students' lifestyle choices. He had never stipulated that I, or any of us, become celibate, and back in San Francisco I had not even considered such a thing. But for the time being, this abstemious state seemed wholly natural. I could not have imagined siphoning off my energies in the way that a sexual bond would have demanded.

Still, I was not strictly without affectionate companionship. Amigo still spent much of each day by my side. There were times when he'd go off exploring, jumping the wall down by the *estero* to roam the jungle, or he'd loaf around in a patch of shade with Maya and her puppies. But if he wasn't around and I so much as thought of him, he'd usually come running. I rarely had to call his name aloud.

Occasionally, I would have an actual conversation with someone other than Anna or Fernando. By chance one morning, as I thought about taking a long, hot walk down the beach to the San Diego bus, I saw a car pulling out of the gate of the adjacent property. I ran over to ask the people in the car if they happened to be headed to La Libertad. They turned out to be our neighbors, Miguel and Maria, an attractive couple in their midthirties. They graciously offered me a ride, and since the day was already scorching, I gratefully accepted, piling into the back of their new black Mercedes beside their three-year-old daughter and two-year-old son. During the twenty-five-minute trip to town, I learned that Miguel and Maria lived most of the year in the capital, San Salvador, and had been schooled in the United States. Both spoke fluent English and were pleased to have a chance to practice it. But to my surprise, the sound of English disturbed me a bit. It seemed somehow harsh compared to Spanish, and more than that, it served to break the spell of wonderment under which I'd been living. The family was warm and welcoming, but I never did spend much time with them after that morning, except for the occasional hello at the beach or a hitchhike into town now and again. Still, it was good to know that kindhearted people were right next door.

If there was one fly in my ointment, it buzzed around only once every four weeks or so, when the full moon had a strange and unhappy effect on the usually gentle Fernando. Why did it affect him so? I know folklore would have it that our *guardián* was sensitive to the moon's pull on him—that we are mostly water, after all, and so we have inner tides. I had also heard that how someone acts during the full moon depends on what is already embedded in his or her mind and emotions, either from this lifetime or from past lives. If true, the moon, at the time of its strongest gravitational pull, was exciting Fernando's deep-seated demons and turning unconscious desires to action.

I also remembered Walt's guidance during our stargazing practices. He'd said to be cautious when gazing into the full moon. "When you do this without being aware, you are open to the energies of other people—good or evil—that are drawing on the full moon for personal power."

Whatever was happening to Fernando, one thing was certain:

out in the wilds of El Salvador, the moon had a radical impact on him.

The first two times Fernando went "lunatic" I tried to ignore it. I said nothing when his shouts woke me at midnight and I peered out from behind my curtains to see him cackling maniacally, circling the courtyard on his rickety bicycle. A month later, I again said nothing when he and his friends broke the still of the night with a whooping dance around a blazing bonfire. But the third time, Anna awoke me to tell me Fernando was threatening the neighbor's *guardián* with Walt's gun. This was no longer irksome mischief; it was genuine danger.

That night, with the dazzling orb illuminating the inky black jungle sky, I tapped into the deepest recesses of my own unconscious and found what I experienced as immediate and palpable guidance from Walt. Incredibly, I summoned up a sense of deep calm, and with it the courage to demand that Fernando surrender the gun to me. Following an inner voice, I put a stop to a horrible scene that might well have ended tragically.

My intervention that night changed many things. It bettered my relationship with Fernando, who treated me with a new level of respect. It empowered me, and allowed me to feel more comfortable in the role for which I'd been chosen. And although I did not know it yet, it turned out to end, once and for all, the cycle of full moon mania at our otherwise peaceful oasis.

More important to me than any of that, however, it seemed to link me to Walt in a profound new way. Since Gurudev had left, I'd felt he'd been sending me messages in subtle ways: the presence or absence of eggs in the hens' nests, the companionable love of Amigo, the powerful waves of calm that would sometimes wash over me as I practiced my prescribed yoga poses. But the night of the gun incident initiated a more direct connection. The voice that guided me that night was palpable and unmistakable. Walt had somehow manifested in my consciousness. When I heard him say, "You must control your own mind or negativity will," it was more than a memory. It was more than asking myself, "What would Gurudev say?" and providing my own answer. It was an in-the-moment communication. I knew with certainty from then on that if I needed Walt he would, in one way or another, be there.

In the aftermath of that revelation, I became more energized than ever, and my zeal seemed to be contagious. The construction work on the unfinished parts of the retreat proceeded at an accelerated pace. The workmen seemed happy and inspired. The hens laid eggs like they were competing for jackpot prizes. I believed that Walt sensed from afar how proud I was of all that was being accomplished, and I looked forward to filling him in.

In the second week of February, shortly after the eventful full moon, I set out to make a telephone call to Walt from the phone company office in La Libertad to tell him about the distressing incident and to get his advice on how best to deal with Fernando in the future. It was, once again, a blazing hot day. The temperature in La Libertad was normally about ten degrees higher than at the retreat, mainly because the stucco of the town's many buildings radiated an oven-like heat. The intensity of the heat I experienced that day was compounded by the fact that I had missed the first bus in San Diego and did not arrive in town until eleven thirty in the morning. The streets were almost empty. A few men were leaning against the walls surrounding the town square, motionless. Even the watermelon vendor, whose business was usually brisk, was nowhere to be seen.

Fortunately, the only air-conditioned building in La Libertad was the phone company. There was a big crowd that day, drawn no doubt by a desire to cool off, and I tried to temper my impatience by repeating my mantra and breathing practice as I stood in a long line—and then sat waiting even longer for the call to be put through by a bored-looking man who couldn't have cared less if I waited all day. When I finally got through to Walt, I told him of Fernando's behavior.

"Michele, you did the right thing. Do not return the gun to Fernando. Keep it safe until I return," Walt said, "I'll be there soon."

"You will? *Wonderful!*" I exclaimed, immediately thrilled and anxious.

"Yes, it's time," he confirmed. "I want to prepare some things for when the first group of students comes down. There is much to be done and you are ready now."

What did he mean by that? I wondered.

"Patience," Walt said, even though I'd said nothing aloud. "I'll be there in two weeks."

The day Walt was due to arrive, Amigo abandoned me to pace back and forth by the gate. Maya soon joined him, and there was no doubt the two loyal dogs sensed exactly what was going on. Part of me felt like pacing back and forth myself I was so eager to greet Walt and to see his reaction to everything that had been accomplished. Instead, I busied myself with last-minute tidying, putting the finishing touches on two weeks' worth of zealous spring-cleaning in which Anna and I had collaborated. In my humble opinion, everything on the property looked splendid. At my request, Fernando had even pulled all the dead branches off the coconut trees, so that even Mother Nature herself was freshened up.

Walt was late. The muggy, late February afternoon turned into a pleasantly warm evening and as it did, even though Walt had still not arrived, my restlessness subsided and a deeper calm than I had ever known began to come over me. Rather than wait nervously and expectantly, as would have been my habit before El Salvador, I went into the meditation room thinking that perhaps I had the day wrong, or that somehow he had been delayed. Rather than feeling disappointed and anxious, I luxuriated in the attitude that all of the preparations had been completed, I had done my duty to the best of my ability, and now life was giving me time to turn inward.

About a half hour into my practice, I felt a distinct shift. I knew the moment Walt's taxi was about to pull up—not just because I could hear Amigo bark but also because I felt the same uplifting spine tingle that I always seemed to experience when Gurudev was nearby. The air itself seemed to shimmer.

Fernando and I both arrived at the gate as Walt paid the driver, but although we greeted him in unison, each of us came bearing a very different mind-set. Fernando was grinning widely, yet I could tell he had his antennae out. He was feeling shame and nervously anticipating Walt's reaction to him in light of the gun episode. I remained amazingly peaceful inside myself, even as I expressed joy and excitement at Gurudev's return. This sensation of tranquil strength was new to me, and yet I observed myself wearing it as though it had always been a part of me. *This must be what true balance feels like,* I thought. *In the midst of the outer excitement, there is a center of pure beingness. In my center, I AM.*

Although Walt Baptiste was not a tall man, he possessed a large barrel chest and muscular frame from years of bodybuilding and intensive yoga practices. His very presence exuded power, conviction and compassion. He always looked neat and put together in clothes that generally had an ethnic flavor, and tonight was no exception. A long strand of large turquoise prayer beads circled his neck, peeking out from under an elegantly handwoven Guatemalan vest. A subtle scent of sandalwood surrounded him. Not looking the slightest bit travel worn from his long journey, Walt greeted Fernando warmly—much to Fernando's apparent relief. Then he turned to greet me, beaming with admiration.

"Congratulations, Michele. You have done a beautiful job both for yourself and for all here."

My heart glowed and I smiled serenely. "Thank you. It's a blessing to have you back with us."

It was then that I remembered my manners. "Are you hungry, Gurudev? Can I get you something?"

"No, thank you, Michele," he replied. "I had something to eat on the plane and it's late."

"What about fresh coco water?"

He lit up. "A pitcher of coco water brought to the house would be perfect. And now I will bid you both good night. We have a busy day tomorrow."

His final words of the evening would become a signature El Salvador good night: "Dream great dreams and live them out in the morning."

At that moment, the peacefulness that I had been experiencing that evening deepened. It stole over me like a mist until it permeated every part of my being and radiated out into the scene unfolding before me. For a perfect moment, I was truly present in all the strength and stillness that my soul possessed. I watched with a profound sense of wonder and gratitude as Fernando followed Walt up the stairs and into his quarters, carrying his two large leather suitcases that seemed to be bursting at the seams with unknown treasures.

The next morning, after Walt came out of his house, I literally had to pry Amigo and Maya loose from their long-lost master, but I finally managed to begin the grand tour. It was odd to be the one showing Walt around, for it hadn't been long since he'd done the same for me. Yet I was pleased to point out the new rooms that had been finished and the structures that had been expanded on my watch. Walt seemed pleased too, and complimented my accomplishments as manager. He enthusiastically agreed that very soon we could begin to fulfill the retreat's mission as a place of respite and renewal for anyone who wanted to make the trip.

In the two weeks Walt stayed, he and I made three trips to the capital city of San Salvador, braving its heavy free-for-all traffic patterns and pollution as we shopped for basic furnishings for the newly finished accommodations. We gathered simple beds, mattresses and table lamps. The trips were hot and exhausting, and we returned with our clothing soaked through with perspiration. Still, it was gratifying to see the retreat transforming from an idea to a reality right before my eyes.

Our other major endeavor during that period was the planting of a sizable garden. Walt had always loved tending gardens, while I had a notorious "black thumb" that instilled fear and trembling in every innocent houseplant I'd ever attempted to nurture. Nevertheless, I mustered all possible optimism and enthusiasm as we turned over the earth on a twenty-foot-by-thirty-foot plot between the gym and the wall by the *estero*.

Walt wanted us to grow as much of our own produce as possible, and to start we planted tomatoes, cucumbers, bell peppers, beets, and radishes, all from seeds. Walt planned to keep everything strictly organic. Pesticides were verboten, so we also planted marigolds to keep aphids away and made a spray of jalapeño peppers and garlic that would serve as a natural pesticide. Though I suspected the biggest danger to our little seeds was actually me, I didn't say so and barely let myself think so. I listened earnestly to Walt's methodical instructions about spraying and weeding and watering everything twice a day, hoping the Divine Mother would come to my rescue.

Though Walt spent a good deal of time alone in meditation or consulting with the workmen, it was thrilling for me to have him around. But it was also challenging. On my own, I'd gotten into certain habits, some of which Walt was determined to undo. Like a frugal housewife, he chided me every time I left a light on in a room I was leaving. In the kitchen, he fussed loudly whenever I spilled water on the floor, which I have to admit I did often, since the sink was set up in such a way that it was almost impossible to not spill water, unless you were totally conscious of your actions all the time. At first, I felt a bit annoyed. Hadn't I done a yeoman's job here overall? Okay, I might be the tiniest bit careless about small, almost inconsequential matters from time to time, but what about the big picture? Then, one night I began to suspect that Walt was actually trying to tell me something more. I'd emerged from the meditation room having deliberately flicked off the light switch before I closed the door behind me. Walt was just outside and looked at me carefully.

"Michele, you didn't turn the light off," he said.

"I thought I did, Gurudev."

"No, you did not," he insisted.

Ha! I thought. *He's flat-out mistaken. I'll show him.*

I opened the door to vindicate myself, anticipating how gracious I'd be in the face of Walt's inevitable apology. Instead, I found the light I had definitely turned off was clearly on. He aimed a piercing gaze at me and said simply, "Be conscious, Michele."

He turned on his heel, leaving me dumbfounded at my own lack of mindfulness. *How could I have left the light on? How? And why was Walt so vigilant about this?* Then it dawned on me that on some level, Walt had to be speaking metaphorically. Back in San Francisco, Walt had mentioned many times the importance of closing off psychic doorways after meditation before going out in public. "You don't just wake up in the morning and run out of the house, do you?" he'd say. "You need to bring your energies out again to meet the energies of the world." He'd taught us to use deep breathing to shift psychic gears, training us to "take the best moment you experienced inside, reach in with your breath, and pull it into your body, into the room, and into your life and affairs."

Here in El Salvador, I'd ignored that discipline. Used to so little company and so few intrusions from the "real world" at large, I'd stopped mindfully transitioning from one state to another. Obviously, this was something Walt had noticed and disapproved of, and I understood why. Someday I would be back in civilization, where it would be more important than ever to set boundaries around my inner and outer states of being. You don't want to walk down a city street with one foot in what is essentially another dimension. In a way, "shutting the light" is a form of spiritual protection. If you leave yourself wide open psychically, all kinds of energies can penetrate—some of them not very beneficial. I had a taste of the consequences a few times during my time at the San Francisco Center when I left the meditation room without bringing my energies out thoroughly. I had hurried down to work in the restaurant and once there, could barely function. Overly sensitive and withdrawn, the only thing I wanted to do was go home and curl up into a little ball. I was basically useless until Colin, noticing me hiding in the back room, saved the day by sending me out to the garden to breathe deeply.

Walt's chiding about my spilling water, I now believed, was a metaphor as well, but one I did not decipher as quickly. As time went on, though, I figured it out. Whenever I was not paying enough attention to my *kriya* work, which moves the energy up the spine to the higher chakras, puddles and dripping faucets and leaky pipes seemed to plague me. The leaks coincided with my leaking *kundalini* energy. Even today, years after Walt left his body and passed on from this world, the same holds true: when I neglect my *kriya* work something around me trickles or dribbles or floods. I truly believe it is Walt's way of reminding me to *bring the energy up.* That's why while most people call a plumber when something's leaking, I take it as a message from the universe to redirect my spiritual energy. Then I call the plumber.

Once it occurred to me that Walt's nagging was actually a teaching, I felt even more honored than before to be with him at the retreat without having to share him with any other students. When he inquired about how my Hatha Yoga practice was going, I was eager to tell him of my progress. I was holding some of my assigned postures, like the bridge and the forward bend, for up to forty-five minutes. And I could do a headstand for a half hour. Walt, to my surprise, told me I should now spend less time in the postures.

"You're achieving the right state of mind more quickly," he said, "and that is the point. You must learn to relax in the *asanas* more quickly for quicker results. You should get the same results in three or five minutes that before took a half hour. Then, go even deeper. Each time, begin your relaxation at the point you left off the last time.

"Besides, I want to add another practice for you to work on."

His new assignment for me was spending an hour a day in a breath-watching practice. "Follow the breath into the nostrils as far as you can follow it, until the two nostrils join inside the head and you sense there is just one passageway," he instructed. "Then follow it out as far as you can follow it."

After an hour of this, I was to focus my attention at the point in the head where the two breath streams had joined, look inside, and add my mantra. One purpose of this was to open up my third eye. "There are more beautiful worlds inside than outside," Gurudev told me. "Use your new energy to really look inside."

As always, I was delighted to be given a new practice by Walt and anxious to try to perfect it after he left. In fact, he was leaving soon, and though I was certainly not looking forward to it, I did flatter myself that I had grown closer to him during this trip. I had spent the kind of quality time with him that most of his students could only dream of and, truth be told, it was beginning to change the dynamics between us. Shopping, dining, swimming, and doing worldly things with my guru caused me to relax the boundaries between teacher and student. In a sense, I forgot whom I was with. I still, of course, was respectful of Walt as teacher, but I forgot the full import of the guru-disciple relationship. I began relating to him more in the human dimension than in the divine dimension, where such a relationship is formed and meant to play out over many lifetimes. Familiarity breeds informality, and my newfound laxity began to show itself in subtle ways—in casual conversation, in the way I would respond to his questions, even in a slight slowing down in my personal practice.

Then, the day before he departed, Walt invited me down for a cooling dip in the ocean. It was late morning and unusually overcast for that time of the year. The ocean looked royal blue, and clouds were moving rapidly across the canvas of the sky. The surf was relatively calm, the waves barely rippled, and it was easy enough to wade out waist deep.

Walt asked me if I had any questions before he left. At that moment I felt like the golden girl. During this trip, Walt had, directly and indirectly, showered me with praise and special attention. He was obviously pleased with my work so far, seemingly in every way. My comfort level with myself was very high and the memory of the Light that I had experienced in his San Francisco yoga class was ever present.

He replied softly, "If you keep practicing the way you've been practicing, you will most certainly get there, Michele. But at this moment you aren't ready to be trusted with that kind of knowledge."

I silently started to protest. *What? Me, not trustworthy? Hadn't I done everything my guru asked, and then some? Aren't I more than ready to take the next step on this journey?*

Suddenly the waves began to whip up with tremendous force, the current whirled around me, and the sky darkened. I looked to Walt for an explanation and was taken aback by the fierce, wild expression on his face. Later, I reread in the Hindu classic the *Bhagavad-Gita* a description of the furious and awesome face of the god Krishna that he unmasked for his student Arjuna to see, and it brought me back to that moment, that expression. Before I could utter a word, Walt thrust his arm below the surface of the water and pulled out a writhing, giant, crimson starfish, nearly two feet in diameter. He raised his arm and set the amazing creature wriggling toward the heavens. Looking at me with a piercing gaze, he threw back his head and, with a booming voice that must have resonated to the far reaches of the cosmos, said, "Look for the star *inside!*"

I was completely overwhelmed by the sight, by the sheer magnificent power of what I was seeing, that I nearly passed out right there in the ocean with the now roiling waves crashing around me. I had never experienced a power of this magnitude before, and I trembled to the core of my being. Even after the moment passed and Walt returned the starfish to the sea, I was stupefied for some time. We walked back to the shore in complete silence, but I knew there was now no need to speak. Never had I seen, nor would I see again, a starfish in the waters of El Salvador. I had received a powerful reminder that Walt was someone and something well beyond the avuncular mentor I'd come to think I was palling around with. I had overstepped my bounds, had puffed up my ego, and sought a shortcut to a destination that could only be reached by a long, hard road. All of that I now saw clearly. What I did not know at that moment, but would soon learn, was just how hard the path before me was about to become.

PART III

Opening the Doors

CHAPTER 13

CINDERELLA

*"The difference between an ordinary man and a sage
is that a sage does not allow anyone to affect his mind
and emotions."*
—SWAMI RAMA, *THE ART OF JOYFUL LIVING*

*A*s I stood in the garden, I couldn't help thinking about
Scarlett O'Hara. I could never forget the iconic scene in which
the *Gone with the Wind* heroine, dazed and starving after General
Sherman's march through Atlanta, pulls a green stalk out
of the ruins of her own garden and gnaws the radish at its end.
Reduced to tears, she famously vows, "I'll never be hungry
again."

Like Scarlett, all I could extract from my plot of earth was a
paltry handful of radishes. Unlike her, I had no rampaging army
to blame. I had only my black thumb. The garden was a failure
despite a month of ministrations, and Walt was coming back any
day now—this time with a group of students. They wouldn't
go hungry, of course, and I could hardly have been expected
to offer up a cornucopia of produce in the month that had
elapsed since the garden was sown. Nevertheless, I was worried
about Walt's reaction. I wanted nothing but more praise from

him, especially in front of others. I consoled myself that some small patches of green, new arrivals over the last few days, were sprouting up here and there. Maybe my horticultural curse was about to lift.

Was everything else in order? For at least the third time that day, I patrolled the grounds and surveyed the state of the retreat with a critical eye. I reassured myself that everything seemed fine. The rooms for the visitors (three would arrive with Walt, including his nineteen-year-old-daughter Devi, and eight more would join them a few days later) were ready and waiting. The kitchen pantry was stocked. The meditation room was swept and prepped. Check, check, check. I allowed myself a self-congratulatory moment.

Things had settled into a groove for me here, or so it seemed. After Walt left the last time, I was so overcome with awe, so bedazzled by the lingering image of that resplendent starfish, that I had renewed with even greater passion my intention to be the perfect manager of this sacred setting. Soon after, though, I'd been waylaid for a few weeks by a bout of illness. I'd succumbed to a low-grade fever and headache and occasionally took to bed, where I dozed to dull the pain behind my eyes. Anna had brought me plain tortillas, which were all I felt like eating, and countless cold compresses. She worried I might have dengue fever, a viral disease spread by mosquitoes throughout the tropics, but I insisted it was just the flu. Because I never had a blood test, I never knew what I'd actually had. Nevertheless, I dragged around and somehow managed to do my chores.

The workmen were still making progress. The animals were healthy. Our supplies, while running low, had sufficed. I credited myself with running a tight ship and settled into a slightly modified managerial routine that was not quite as frenetic as before. I was more willing to delegate responsibilities, as I told myself any capable manager would be. And, to my eye, that had seemed to pay off.

But my eye was not the guru's eye.

No sooner did Walt arrive than he started noticing all of the things I had neglected to observe. The pool was cloudy and needed backwashing.

"Michele," Walt said, "the pool should be clear. Didn't you notice the green tinge to the water?" I hadn't, but he was right.

Grime had collected in the grout between the kitchen tiles.

"Michele, didn't you notice the gunk?" I hadn't, but it was true.

Needless to say, the garden was another sore spot.

"Michele, you see these?" Walt said, pointing to the outcropping of shoots I'd considered a promising sign. "They're weeds."

I was mortified to have disappointed Gurudev, and so eager to make everything right that I practically tripped all over myself to do so. When Walt commented that the workmen had not made as much progress this month as he had hoped for, I immediately jumped in to try to make amends.

"I'll talk to them right away," I offered. "I've been too soft with them. I apologize."

But Walt said no. "You haven't been too soft, Michele. You are too officious. I can hear it in your tone. You're behaving like the queen. You rule rather than inspire and encourage. With the workmen and with Fernando, too. You had too many little things for him to do and neglected the important things. You should let the workers do their work and allow more freedom within the structure. Don't forget what this place is about. It is about love."

I had *not* forgotten! Or had I? With every observation Walt made, I became less sure of myself. My anxiety led to more carelessness, and soon it seemed like I was digging myself deeper. One afternoon, I was so determined to help clean up speedily after lunch that I stuffed a blender into a high kitchen cupboard just to get it out of the way. The next day, Walt opened the cupboard and the blender clattered to the floor. It would have crashed onto his head if he hadn't ducked quickly. He said not a word, but he didn't have to. I knew what he was thinking: *How easy do you think it will be to find a new blender in the middle of the jungle?*

Why Walt said nothing about having to dodge a falling kitchen appliance was, no doubt, because others were around when it happened. He always saved his comments and corrections for when we were alone, and for this I was infinitely grateful. Nevertheless, his daughter Devi and the couple who had accompanied her down, an old San Francisco friend of mine named Jon and his friend Karen, had witnessed the incident. This was enough to make me even more self-conscious, even though Jon and Karen, both talkative by nature, had the good grace to pretend nothing much had happened and barely missed a beat in their conversation.

Later that day, when he caught me alone, he furiously reprimanded me for going unconscious. "Michele," he commanded, "you are not to concentrate on yoga postures so much anymore. You must concentrate on the things you are doing on this plane. Carry out your duties with your mind one hundred percent there, and find ease in each situation quickly and with joy."

By the time the other eight students arrived at the retreat, I was an emotional Jell-O mold. I may have looked quite presentable on the outside, but inside I was quivering, wondering what I'd neglected to do or done poorly that Walt would pinpoint next. The infusion of what, for me, was a massive amount of company after months of contented isolation, didn't help me feel any more stable, even though most of those who came were familiar faces. To escape both Walt's scrutiny and the cacophony of English-speaking voices, I spent a great deal of time off by myself pulling weeds, cleaning the pool, and scrubbing the kitchen.

I was vigilant about maintaining my practices too, though determined not to let them interfere with my managerial duties. I tried rising even earlier than usual to begin my yoga, meditation, and *kriya* work. Walt had always said that the hour between 3:00 and 4:00 a.m. was ideal for meditation, because the body is quiescent and the mind is open and uncluttered. Habitually a late sleeper, this interlude was foreign territory to me, but I decided to give it a try. Although rousing myself at that hour required herculean effort, I did my best to throw back the bedsheet and tap into my inner world long before the roosters crowed in the outer one.

Sitting alone in the meditation room before dawn, I struggled to quiet my mind. In my clearest and most expansive moments, it came to me that perhaps I was overreacting. Walt had never raised his voice to me, so why did I feel that I was being "yelled at"? He never criticized me in front of others, so why was I feeling humiliated? And everything he said about the buildup of weeds and gunk and grime was, in fact, so. Even though on one level I thought I was doing my best, I looked at myself honestly and had to admit that I did have a tendency to compromise my best and slide backward. So why was I feeling picked on? I decided I needed to get past my reactions and start looking at what message Walt might be sending me. After a while, I concluded that Walt's drawing my attention to gunk and grime buildup was, in fact, my guru's latest metaphor. *Eureka!* I thought. *He is trying to tell me that my own energy is stagnant.*

Convinced I had unlocked the secret, I redoubled my efforts at *kriya* practice. The great yoga masters teach that *kriya* work, the various esoteric practices of channeling the energy that lies coiled at the base of the spine, serves not only to liberate the soul, but also to free the body-mind of toxic buildup by unleashing a reservoir of additional *prana*. It is an elixir that works by saturating decaying cells with undecayable light. But beyond enlarging consciousness and prolonging life, Kriya Yoga, if done daily with the right guidance and right attitude, is said to dramatically speed up one's karma. The self-realization that might take a million years of lifetimes to attain could be achieved in one lifetime alone by a disciplined practitioner of *kriya*. We enter each incarnation with *samskaras*, subtle impression of past incarnations, emblazoned upon our body and mind. *Kundalini* is the only force powerful enough to cut through this karmic buildup, like ammonia cutting through—aha!—kitchen grease.

I remembered something that Yogananda wrote in his *Autobiography of a Yogi*: "One thousand *kriyas* practiced in eight and a half hours gives the yogi, in one day, the equivalent of one thousand years of natural evolution." I did the math and decided to work up to this number as quickly as I could. By my calculations, I might be enlightened before I turned thirty-five! This obviously must be what Walt had in mind.

Surprisingly, though, my revelation, and my accelerated attentions to my spinal column, had little impact on Walt's disposition toward me. He kept finding traces of grunge and muck; I kept scrubbing. Nothing changed. No matter how long or hard I practiced, I was a spiritual Cinderella.

Then, a few days before Walt and our visitors were due to

leave, Gurudev asked me to walk with him. We walked near the ocean to the glorietta, a large umbrella-like structure made of woven palm fronds that provided shelter from the sun. He motioned for me to sit beside him under it and proceeded to pull out of his knapsack several strands of large *rudraksha* seeds from India. *Rudraksha* seeds, classically used by yogis as prayer beads or *malas*, are said to contain all of the five elements of nature: space, air, water, fire, and earth. I was elated to sit with him and quietly string our *malas* together onto strong fishing wire. Sharing this simple yet deeply meaningful task lightened my heart. Because the beads were rather large, we decided to use 54 for each of our *malas* rather than the traditional 108, which meant I would count each bead twice around as I recited my mantra. As we neared the end of our stringing, Walt fished around in his backpack and pulled out a few coral beads and a beautiful amber bead. "These are for you to add to your prayer beads," he said, his eyes sparkling. "They are from Tibet."

I was so, so happy. At that moment I felt that all my inadequacies had been forgiven, and I said as much in a profuse rush of gratitude and self-abnegation. "I'm so sorry about my second-rate performance, Gurudev. I will do my very best for you and for the retreat. I will be aware of buildup and will do my best to keep all the energies flowing. And I'm practicing my *kriya* work as you asked."

But Walt looked stern again. "Michele, this is not about what I want."

"It isn't?"

"Of course not. How could it be? Your problem is that you don't yet really trust yourself. You were thrown off balance completely when all of us arrived. You lost your center. And you lost it because you are far too dependent on other people's judgments of you. You think you took action, but all you did was react."

"But I just want to please you."

"Being pleased with yourself because you think others are pleased with you is just the empty satisfaction of ego."

Now I was really confused. Walt looked deeply into my eyes as he continued in a soft but serious tone. "There is a distinction between an ordinary person and a yogi. A yogi draws strength from inside. She does not react to praise or criticism. She does not allow any other individual to influence whether she accepts herself. That is a surrender of power. When you give up your power, your center, that is when you go unconscious and become what you call 'second-rate.'"

Although part of me understood, part of me still groped for a solution. I sought a quick fix I could offer up to my guru so he would see I was determined to reinvent myself as a true yogi.

"I see," I said. "Well, won't my *kriya* practice help me get stronger inside?"

Walt shook his head. "*Kriya* work, kitchen work—for you right now it's all the same. There is no benefit to anything you do unless you do it because you feel it is the right thing. Only then will you do anything the right way."

He stopped for a moment and looked at me deeply, as though he were looking into my heart.

"Michele," he said kindly, "don't worry so much about being loved. Be more of what love is."

With that, Walt began walking back toward his house, and I fell silently in step with him. I was trying so hard to process everything he had said. Maybe to some people his message would not have been such a cosmic news flash, but I had spent my life as an inveterate people-pleaser. The idea that I should not react to others' opinions of me, or expend any of my energy getting everyone to like me, was freeing and terrifying at once.

And so I started repeating to myself my new mantra: *Don't react, don't react.*

But another thought impression was speaking even louder in my head: *Maybe I'm not really capable of this.*

As if in answer, Walt told me one more thing. "When I leave," he said, "Devi will be staying on for a little while—and while she does, she'll be taking over as manager. Help her where you can."

My introduction to Walt's daughter Devi was seeing her perform with Magaña's troupe. She was an astonishingly gifted dancer, lithe and graceful, and like any natural talent, she made even her most difficult maneuvers seem entirely effortless. In San Francisco, the two of us crossed paths repeatedly as Devi came and went from dance to yoga classes and from Magaña's exotic clothing boutique, where she helped out part-time. Although I liked and admired her, we were nearly ten years apart in age and were not close friends. Now she had my job.

Once Walt and the others left, Devi and I were in the somewhat awkward situation of having to switch roles. She was to check on the workmen, consult with Anna about the housekeeping, and go to town for supplies. I was to . . . what? I wasn't entirely certain.

Remembering what Walt had said—to not judge myself in relation to others, to not react—I tried mightily to regard my new circumstances not as proof of my failure as a manager, but as a gift of time in which to further my practices. In fact, it was something of a relief to be able to focus on my yoga and meditation without the many other day-to-day obligations I'd been used to fulfilling. I reorganized my schedule, aware that if I did not stick to one, in spite of these changes, I might lapse into mediocrity. And I still spent a lot of time in the happy company of Amigo, who offered me his usual unconditional adoration regardless of the shift in my status.

Toward Devi I had mixed feelings. I genuinely liked her, but still being far from the perfectly dispassionate yogi, I felt jealous of her as well. She was exquisitely beautiful, and next to her I felt ugly and fat. I tried hard not to show this—so hard that at times I think I overwhelmed her with my strained attempts to befriend her. The two of us were unfailingly polite to one another and took the high road as we tried to figure out the best way (or the least emotionally clumsy way) to relate. But despite a bit of approach-avoidance dynamics, we did a good job of finding the right distance from one another: not too far, not too near.

After the first week or so, our routine was more or less set, and I was feeling better about it all. Walt's talk under the glorietta had left me stronger, but humbled. I knew there was internal work to be done and I set my course. Besides, I knew that Devi's time at the retreat was limited, since she soon would head back to the States to continue her teaching. Perhaps I would reassume my management duties shortly. In any case, I was still happy to be here, still steeped in the warm glow of my precious paradise.

But paradise also had changes to go through.

The rainy season had arrived a few weeks earlier, and although we only had a few storms, so far they were dramatic. The earth shook with the loudest crackling thunder I had ever heard in my life and, hour after hour, sheets of rain fell from the heavens as if from a giant bucket. All of nature went on high alert. The birds went wild with laughter and excitement; the dogs found shelter under the veranda near the kitchen door, curling up in fetal positions. The animals on the other side of the property hid in their respective shelters. The trees and plants, designed to survive the pummeling, usually looked better for it afterward, although there were often mounds of branches and debris left behind. Once each storm passed, more often than not we were left without electricity for at least one day, and sometimes as long as three.

But with the rains came a welcome relief. The humidity, which had built to an almost unbearable crescendo, lessened and was replaced with a welcomed coolness. The plants, which were beginning to look worn and listless, now stood tall and vibrant.

One crystal clear June morning, after a rainy, windy night, we woke up to the air alive with *prana*. Devi and I were preparing a light breakfast in the kitchen, feeling fresh and happy, when we heard a car pull up. We ran to the gate just in time to see Matthew helping an attractive brunette out of a taxi.

"Matthew," Devi exclaimed, "what a wonderful surprise!"

Matthew was grinning from ear to ear as he introduced us to his bride, Joanne.

Excitement and congratulations filled the air as Devi and I took turns showering the couple with questions, eager to hear news from home.

"How long will you be with us?" I innocently asked.

"I'm not sure," he answered. "Joanne is pregnant and we are planning on returning home in time for her to have the baby in the States."

Joanne smiled beatifically.

I was stunned beyond words, and my futile attempt to remain calm and composed did not register in my outer demeanor. Sensing my confusion, Matthew quickly pulled an envelope out of his pocket and handed it to me. My name was boldly inscribed in Walt's handwriting on the front. I opened it slowly.

Dear Michele,

Your time in El Salvador is up. You will be going home in four days. You are needed here in San Francisco and we look forward to seeing you at the Center again. I have enclosed your airline ticket. I wish you a safe and peaceful journey.

Gratefully,
Walt Baptiste

CHAPTER 14

THE RAZOR'S EDGE

"If joy were ceaseless here in this world, would man ever desire another?"

—PARAMAHANSA YOGANANDA,
AUTOBIOGRAPHY OF A YOGI

*A*h, June in San Francisco. If you've never experienced it, you'd make the mistake that so many tourists make and, naïvely packing shorts and tank tops, prepare to hang off a streetcar and soak up some California rays. But if you have experienced it, you'd know why they call the gray damp that shrouds the city "June gloom." And you'd certainly agree with Mark Twain's famous observation, "The coldest winter I ever spent was a summer in San Francisco." The Richmond district, where the Baptiste Yoga Center was located, is notorious for fog, and the misty curtain of the solstice hangs especially heavy. It didn't do much to help my state of mind as I struggled to readjust to city life after what I initially thought of as my expulsion from Eden.

In the first few weeks after my unexpected return from El Salvador, I often felt I was on a foreign planet made of cement. The only thing that lightened my mood was the sight of a tree optimistically poking out of a concrete sidewalk. "*That* is real," I would tell myself. It was not so much that everything else felt unreal; it was more that I felt totally dislocated from my own personal reality.

Suddenly, it seemed to me that everyone in America dressed like kings and queens. Their leather and lace stood in stark contrast to the old, worn cotton of the native people who had comprised my recent community. Walking down the streets of the city, I was overwhelmed by the sheer numbers of shops filled with extravagant baubles beckoning me to consume, consume, consume. Desire to own things, an emotion that I had not experienced during my many months in El Salvador, reared its familiar head.

How curious, I thought, gazing into the shop windows, *that I don't experience the feeling of desire and need until I see an object presented to me in an enticing manner.* I wondered, *Am I being manipulated, or is this outer scenario simply triggering what already lies within me?*

As much as I could manage it I went to the beach, where I could look out over the vast sea, tune into the sound of the waves, and try to reconnect with that part of myself that resonated with El Salvador. But still, this was not *my* beach. Where were my coconut trees swaying in the breeze? Where were the miles of sparkling diamond sand? Where oh where was the tropical heat? Above all, where was the silence?

Everywhere, people were talking and talking about—it seemed to me—*absolutely nothing.* The chatter pervaded the streets, the parks, the stores, and, most noticeably to me, the Hungry Mouth restaurant, where I was working once again. As I careened between crowded tables, trying to keep my orders straight amidst the incessant *blah blah* of idle observations and gratuitous gossip, I kept wondering—not very charitably, I'll admit—*Why doesn't everybody just shut up? They don't actually have anything to say!*

Would this too pass? Of course, I kept reminding myself. Of course it would. *Just be here now.* I had made so much progress in El Salvador, had grown so much calmer, become more grounded and capable. But now I felt myself sliding backwards, feeling overwhelmed, and constantly forgetting to "turn out the light." My energy was low and I was exhausted. After I'd been back for about two weeks, Walt pinpointed the problem.

One night, at the end of a yoga class, he'd described my evident fatigue as burnout. "You're short-circuiting, Michele," he'd said. "Your mind is going back to old habits, old conditioning. You're responding to things in ways that are no longer true for you." He was not unkind about it—in fact, he was extremely kind and welcoming to me since I'd come home, reiterating how much I was "needed here"—he was just very patiently stating a fact. The fact was, I was caught between worlds.

"Remember, the goal of the yogi is to be well and at home no matter the outer circumstance. Non-preference is one of the cornerstones of yoga. A true yogi is equally comfortable living in a palace or in a one-room hut," Walt went on with great affection. "I want you to be happy and well within yourself. I know you long for the tropics, but enjoy and appreciate your time here as well. Be well, Michele."

I'd been trying, but it wasn't easy. As soon as I'd landed at the San Francisco airport, plunked down amidst an ear-splitting barrage of English and a crush of hurried countrymen I suddenly thought of as "those Americans," I'd had to acknowledge to myself that for as long as I'd been in El Salvador, I'd had a deep-seated, unspoken fear of having to leave. Now it was time to deal with that fear. But since Walt was being loving and patient with me, I tried to be loving and patient with myself. Even in those tender years I knew it was infinitely easier to feel at one with the universe when you're sitting solo on a mountaintop than when you're immersed in the loose ends of daily life. I set myself the goal of grabbing hold of the best and strongest part of myself that emerged in El Salvador and building on it back in the city. *But take it easy,* I counseled myself. *Don't rush into the world too quickly.*

Just as I had in my first years in San Francisco, I decided to take advantage of the support and protection of the Center. In addition to my shifts at the restaurant, I began working at Magaña's Bazaar Boutique, which had grown quite successful as unique and colorful bohemian clothing became increasingly mainstream. Years before, the store had been the first to introduce tie-dye, and Magaña was still uncannily ahead of the fashion curve. The Baptistes' world travels contributed to a collection of antique Afghani clothing and museum-quality jewelry. The emporium drew people of all ages and from all walks of life who wanted to indulge a hankering for a spangled peasant shirt or a flowing silk caftan.

The shop also offered essential oils, aromatherapy candles, New Age music, and crystals. Magaña was particularly advanced in her understanding and teaching of the power of crystals and gemstones in physical, mental, and emotional healing, and often employed them in her yoga classes to shift energy. "Everything in the universe is vibration," she reminded us. "The refined vibration of crystals and gemstones and their respective colors can reorganize the vibrations of our subtle bodies—the aura of energy that surrounds us—while creating subtle shifts in our mental and physical bodies."

Working in the boutique provided me with plenty of time to experiment with a variety of crystals, holding them and meditating with them. Soon, I became sensitive to their individual energies. Some were so strong that I could feel them pulsating when I enclosed them in my hand. Others pulsed faintly but perceptibly.

Any doubts that I might have entertained regarding crystal power were erased one Saturday morning after Magaña's yoga class. I stayed on after the class to savor the delicious inner tranquility, and when I finally opened my eyes I was completely alone in the yoga temple room. My state of peace was marred slightly by an awareness of my sore left forefinger, on which a minor cut had become infected and stubbornly refused to heal. My gaze fell on a three-foot-high amethyst cathedral crystal on the altar. It was open at the front but with sides and a back that gave it a room-like appearance. Without thinking, I got up from my mat and walked directly to the amethyst, sticking my hurt finger into the opening for a few minutes. When I retracted it, to my amazement there was a noticeable lightening of its angry red wound. By the end of the day, I could barely see where the cut had been. From then on I was an avid promoter of crystals, encouraging our customers to give them a try.

Despite my conflicted thoughts about American consumerism, the boutique's eclectic offerings and open-minded clientele cheered me, as did Magaña herself. One of those petite, compact women who cast a vast and radiant aura, Magaña was a true force of nature. It was small wonder that she had captured Walt's heart at first glance when they met. Their courtship was a whirlwind, but it was hard to imagine any other way to win the heart of this diminutive dynamo. Had he waited, she might have whirled away.

For my first two years at the Center, before going to El Salvador, I thought of myself as "a Walt Baptiste student" who occasionally attended his wife's classes. But this summer, with Walt traveling back and forth to El Salvador and often gone for weeks at a time, I took all the classes I could from her. She taught two yoga classes and four dance classes a week, and as I spent more and more time in her presence, I felt as if her feminine energy was leading me through new doors. Magaña's yoga classes were inspirational, and as colorful as her clothing. She created an atmosphere of joy by augmenting the postures with carefully chosen musical selections and devotional readings. But beyond this, every class was infused with her contagious *joie de vivre*. When I finished one of her classes, I emerged lighter and brighter and filled with a sense of magic. And I often thought of the words she used so often to end a session: "Stay on the beam of light. Don't let anyone pull you from it."

Staying on the beam of light is what I tried to do every day. It was a tricky balancing act, but my practice and my spiritual community served as a net. I made a conscious effort to not resist my reentry, but rather to flow with it, and to make the most of my time back in the "nest." It was quite a period of adjustment for me, and also a tremendous lesson in the workings of the mind. Watching the ebb and flow of different aspects of my consciousness emerging without overreacting to each was a practice in itself. We think we are the same person every day, but we are not. As Walt always said, we are reborn each moment. When I paid attention, I saw for myself this was true.

When I wasn't taking classes or working at the Center, I was often hanging out with a diverse group of friends who also used the Center as a hub. I became closer than I'd been in the past with some of the regulars. One was John—or Big John, as he was fondly called—who, to this day, strikes me as hands-down the funniest human being I have ever met. Big John worked in the gym and the health food store with Norman. He was six foot five, devilishly cute, and an incorrigible flirt—in a goofy and hilarious sort of way. One day he was trying to show me how "ripped" he had gotten from weight lifting, so he tore open his shirt, which he apparently thought was the one that snapped shut, and I desperately tried to keep a straight face as its buttons popped off and fell, one by one, to the floor. John was devoted to exploring metaphysical experiences, but he was also devoted to women—mostly to one in particular: the prima ballerina of the San Francisco Ballet, who was a regular in the restaurant and health food store. The dancer clearly had a boyfriend, though, so Big John pined for her in silence—literally swooning into our arms each time she sweetly bade him good-bye and floated out the door.

I also grew close to Bob, a former member of the chart-topping Jay and the Americans and a fantastic guitar player and songwriter. Along with another guitarist named Bill, a woman who was a pianist and opera singer, and a few others, we began playing together, with me on flute. Walt had written the lyrics for several original spiritual songs, and also selected a few poems from mystics like Kabir, a fifteenth-century Indian poet, and assigned one to each one of us to put to music. At Walt's request, we met five mornings a week for an hour to rehearse together and teach one another the songs. They became the Songs of the Teachings, and we would have concerts and chanting before the Center's Saturday morning meditation session, which was open to the public. One of my favorite songs is music set to a Kabir poem:

Infinite is the grace of the Guru
Infinite is the Good he has done
Infinite eyes he gave to me
To see infinity.

Not all my socializing took place at the Center. Some nights

Bob and I and Herman, the carpenter who had offered me a job as a sander when I first came to the city years back, went out for margaritas. I had been completely abstemious in El Salvador, and at first I wondered if the convivial pastime of social drinking would interfere with my ongoing quest for spiritual fulfillment. But as if in answer, Walt spent much of a class explaining to us why he, unlike many spiritual teachers, didn't prohibit occasional worldly indulgences.

"Some of you ask me if you can eat meat, if you can have a drink, if you can develop a relationship with this one or that one. What is alright? It's simple. Whatever doesn't make you forget your true nature as a spiritual being is alright. Most of us have certain things that *do* make us forget, but those triggers are different for everyone—and sometimes different for the same person at different times. That is the challenge. Know what keeps you remembering and know what stops you from doing so. Know thyself. You have freedom, and you also have responsibility. On the spiritual path, you are walking a very fine line—the razor's edge."

Fortunately for me, the occasional tequila and lime juice cocktail did not seem to impair my spiritual balance. I knew myself well enough to know I was more apt to lose myself in, say, a romantic infatuation, so that was one area where I continued to abstain.

In all, my life back in the city became richer than I had imagined it could be, but in material riches I still had little interest. I was managing to save some money, but I never did look for an apartment of my own. When I first arrived from El Salvador, I house-sat for a girlfriend of mine, whose business often took her out of town. Soon after, I house-sat for her boyfriend, a journalist who had landed an assignment touring with the

Rolling Stones. My house-sitting stints didn't always line up
back to back, though, so Walt offered me a room at the Center
to use whenever I needed. It was not too unusual an arrange-
ment. The building was full of habitable nooks and crannies,
provided you were willing to shower at the public pool down
the street, and both Norman and Herman lived there full time.
My room, about fourteen by ten feet, was upstairs behind the
reception desk and adjacent to the meditation room. It was
entered via two sets of sliding doors. A former office of Walt's,
the room now contained a bed and a few other furnishings
along with various pieces of artwork. Some of the art was made
by Walt, including several sculptures, and some of the art was
of Walt, including an eight-foot-tall painting of Gurudev with
light radiating out of his solar plexus. I spent more than a little
time contemplating that painting.

As June gave way to late summer and foggy gloom gave way
to clearer days, readjustment got progressively easier for me. But
I was still confused as to why Walt yanked me out of El Salvador
the way he did. One day, I decide to ask Norman about it.

"I'm not unhappy here anymore," I said, "or at least I can say
I have many happy moments. But, Norman, I still want to know,
what did I do *wrong*?"

"What makes you think you did anything wrong?" he asked
calmly.

"I thought I was doing a good job, but if I was, why didn't
Walt let me keep on doing it?"

"What good would that have done you?"

"Well, it would have let me stay where I was."

"Why should you want to stay where you are? How does
that help you?"

"You mean Walt did this to help me? Help me what?"

"Michele," Norman said patiently, "first of all, you know deep down that everything the Guru does in relation to you is helpful. I know you know that or you wouldn't be here. As for what he helped you with, it's all about balance. Walt moved you from community to solitude to community. Don't you see why?"

"Because you shouldn't go too far in one direction or the other?"

Norman smiled. I had obviously answered my own question, albeit with some skillful prodding. Suddenly, Walt's motives seemed obvious. It was brilliant, really. His teachings were all about balance. When I went off-kilter he would provide me with the environment to regain the balance between material and spiritual, between inner and outer. His intention was to teach all of us to be true yogis who could be successful in the material world without compromising spiritual practice. My stint back in San Francisco was yet another opportunity to walk the razor's edge.

But still, I had another question.

"Norman, I get it. I really do. But I still wish Walt had told me this at the time he called me home. He seemed so critical of me the last time we were together in El Salvador. He was so severe. Why?"

This time Norman was cryptic. "Read the lives of the saints and sages."

"Okay, sure," I agreed, "but give me a hint, will you?"

He sighed and told me, "The ego has to be shaken to its foundation for it to be rebuilt stronger than before. It happens several times, some say seven times, on the path."

Seven times! It was hard to wrap my brain around.

"Why didn't you want to tell me, Norman? Did you think I'd give up?"

"Oh, no," he said. "That's not it at all. But I'm trying to be more careful about giving spiritual advice. There is a cosmic law that says whenever you teach someone a spiritual principle, you will be the first one tested. Life tests us to make sure that we are up to it within ourselves."

Dear, dear Norman. In the years that have passed since he uttered these words, I have come to appreciate how entirely true they are. I was grateful to him then, and remain even more grateful now, for all the times he went out on a limb for me, and in doing so, invited the universe to present him with a pop quiz.

Once I understood more about the meaning of Walt's summoning me to San Francisco, I began to understand something else as well: sooner or later, I would be going back to El Salvador. It was just a matter of time. A much calmer part of myself began to emerge—almost as serene as I had sometimes felt at the retreat—and I believe it showed. At the end of August, Walt returned from a trip that had lasted several weeks. He gave me a great big hug and said, "It's been a long time since I've seen you." Something about the way he said it, and the way he looked at me, made me think he wasn't talking about his recent absence. He was referring to the real me he knew was "in there"—centered and spiritually connected. A few days later he said, "Michele, it astonishes me how much you have grown in a year."

Hooray! I was as good as on my way.

Ah, but not yet. August ended and September slowly unfurled. Walt indicated I'd be going back to the retreat, but he didn't say when. My eagerness turned briefly to agitation, but then something inside me shifted again. September in San Francisco was typically crisp and bright. I reveled in the company of my spiritual family. I spent hour upon hour in the meditation room, remembering to "turn out the light." In short, I decided to enjoy myself, to enjoy this home.

Then, in early October, I took a yoga class with Walt, and he talked about the importance of how we felt in the postures. "The question to ask," he said, "is, *are you well within yourself?* It's not about how good you look; it's about how well you are." It struck home for me. I'd spent so much of my life putting on a good show outwardly, but being insecure inwardly. Yet, lately I felt confident and well on the inside and comfortable with what surrounded me. I had the sense that I could stay where I was with complete contentment.

So the next day—of course!—Walt told me I would be going back to El Salvador on the twentieth of November, almost a year to the day since the first time I had gone. It seemed to me that being content with what I had was a prerequisite for moving on.

Once again, I packed up my meager belongings and called my parents to tell them I'd be leaving the country. This time, I was surprised by their reaction. Was it really safe to go back to El Salvador now? What about the political unrest, the guerilla activity, the government crackdown that they'd been reading about in the newspaper? I have to confess I knew very little about these things, but nevertheless, I assured them everything would be just fine. How could it not be?

Little did I know that political dangers were the least of my worries, and that within three months I would be fighting a different kind of battle for my life.

CHAPTER 15

NO STONE UNTURNED

*"The conscious mind within ourselves can guide matter . . .
It's possible to change millions and millions of cells in one
moment of powerful intensity."*

—WALT BAPTISTE

El Salvador, 1978

"Señorita, Michele. Señorita Michele." From deep inside the cavernous darkness, I heard the words far above calling me over and over. I tried to resist, but the repetition of my name was insistent. As I slowly began swimming to the surface of consciousness, I half expected to see Anna at my window. But no, this was a man's voice.

My lids flickered open. In the semidarkness of the unfamiliar room, a young man in a white coat was leaning over me solicitously, blowing cigarette smoke into my face. My confusion was apparent.

"Michele, I am Dr. Hernandez, the night physician here. You have been in our private hospital for three days, and you are a very sick woman." He spoke English relatively well, but with a strong accent.

The odor of the smoke was nauseating, and I weakly begged him to put his cigarette out. He did, muttering, "Ah ha" in a knowing way. "Patients with hepatitis cannot tolerate cigarette smoke."

Hepatitis?

Recent memories came tumbling back. The week of high tropical fevers, a trip from the retreat to a free clinic in La Libertad confirming that I did not have malaria but in fact had a severe case of hepatitis A, a viral infection of the liver. My semiconscious taxi ride into San Salvador, my fellow yogi Bob imploring the driver to deliver me to a decent hospital. After that not much—only sleep and more sleep.

"You are being fed intravenously, but tomorrow we will be bringing you food. What do you feel like eating?" The mere thought of eating anything was nauseating, but I told him I might be able to tolerate plain yogurt with honey.

Once the doctor left, I looked around the simple room and thankfully realized I was alone. I tried to objectively scan my body and sum up my current physical state. It was not good. Besides feeling nauseous from the residue of the cigarette smoke, I ached all over. I could barely move. My thoughts were thick and dull. I, Michele, was trapped inside a war-torn vehicle.

I vaguely remembered a consoling passage from the great Hindu spiritual classic *the Bhagavad-Gita*: "That which pervades the entire body you should know to be indestructible. No one is able to destroy that imperishable soul."

I am not this body. I am not this body. I am not this body. I reminded myself, *The body is a vehicle for the spirit. I am untouched.* This spiritual teaching soothed my soul, but it did not seem to alleviate my acute physical misery. Nevertheless, I kept repeating it, and within moments I drifted back into the welcomed solace of sleep.

My hospital stay lasted for two weeks. Because this was a private hospital, it was immaculate, and the staff was caring and competent. But it was also expensive, particularly because hepatitis patients are extremely contagious and require their own rooms.

Bob, who had been staying at the retreat when I'd taken ill, and to whom I appeared to owe my life, had called Walt to let him know what had happened. Shortly after Bob had arrived in El Salvador, I'd fallen ill. Day after day I'd felt more feverish and fatigued. At night, my fever would get so high that I was delirious. When I got sicker and sicker, Bob worried that I had malaria and insisted we go to La Libertad's free medical clinic. The female doctor there took one look at me, handed me a mirror and said, in Spanish, "Look at your eyes. They're bright yellow." Jaundice is a classic sign of hepatitis, signifying an inflamed and impaired liver. The doctor gave me a list of things to do, including an instruction to avoid fats. In my confused state, and with my Spanish being rusty from my six months out of the country, I got this completely backward, thinking she'd said to *eat* fats. Back at the retreat later that night, a handful of butter cookies sent me over the edge.

"I'm dying," I told Bob. This did not feel like hyperbole. I'd had to lie down in the back seat of a cab as we made for help in San Salvador.

After Bob told Walt what had happened, Walt immediately phoned me from San Francisco, insisted that I not leave the hospital until he arrived, and promised he would take care of everything. As it turned out, I needed every minute of the two-week hospital stay. Day by day, slowly, my healing progressed and, finally, I was able to get out of bed and situate myself in a lovely, small garden on the hospital grounds where I practiced gentle yoga postures, did breathing exercises, and played my flute, which Bob had kindly delivered to me after week one.

～

True to his word, Walt, along with Magaña, arrived to take me back to the retreat where I could continue to recuperate. Once there, I humbly realized that the old adage was true: no one is indispensable. Everything was running smoothly. Bob assured me he had taken over my duties. I was not to worry about a thing and take the time to rest completely. There was still genuine concern about contagion, however. Walt and Magaña had arrived with a group of students, and I was placed in semi-quarantine for everyone's protection. I'd have to wash my own sheets and dine alone for several weeks more.

During my convalescence, I had ample time to review the months leading up to my illness. In the teachings of yoga, expectations are to be avoided. We set ourselves up and then are often disappointed when what we anticipate and what actually occurs do not match. Nothing about this second trip to El Salvador was matching my expectations. Everything had been different from the moment my plane touched down at the country's shiny new international airport four months ago.

The first thing I'd noticed was the number of soldiers at the airport, with machine guns in tow. Clearly, the political climate was changing. Next, when I arrived at the retreat, I was introduced to a new *guardián*, Carlos, a former member of the Salvadoran army and a crack horseman. Walt told me that Fernando had been sent away—gone to live with his mother in Playa San Diego—because his drinking had gotten out of control. Unlike the docile (when sober) Fernando, Carlos was extremely macho. To take orders from a woman did not come easily to him. But with political instability hovering in the background, he was a wise choice as protector of the property. Carlos' wife, Gloria, and their two young girls also became part of retreat life.

There were also exciting new additions to the property. New stables were occupied by two horses: Lucero, a strong white stallion whose name meant "Light," and Naranja, "Orange," a sweet chestnut mare. One of my jobs was to ride the horses daily, and as we did not yet have saddles, I learned to ride bareback using only reins. It was exhilarating to ride along the breaking waves with Naranja. Lucero was still beyond my reach and I left him to Carlos, who rode him proudly.

Another new development was the construction of a pyramid on the grounds. Walt was quiet about the project, which had begun in my absence, and had the work on it stopped whenever he left the country. He alluded to it now and then, but for the most part the pyramid was shrouded in mystery. Needless to say, I couldn't wait to find out more about it.

Since I'd returned here from San Francisco, I'd yet to be really alone. I arrived with Walt and Magaña, and the day after they left for the States, my friend Bob and another yoga student, Kate, arrived. Bob was to stay for six months and Kate for two months. As it turned out, it was a blessing that I'd had their companionship when I got sick. Now they, along with the Baptistes, made it clear that I should take all the time I needed to recover.

Since arriving at my hospital bedside, Walt showered me with love and concern. He watched me carefully as we walked to his car and drove back to the retreat. It must have been obvious to him that I was still very weak. Nevertheless, I fully expected to bounce back quickly. It never occurred to me that my recovery would take much longer than I'd hoped. But so much, once again, for expectations.

When we arrived at the retreat, Walt personally helped me to the door of my small room. "I am very sorry that this has happened to you, Michele," he said. "For the next several weeks I want you to completely rest. The liver is a vital organ and your nutrition is now more important than ever. You must be aware of every bite that you put in your mouth. It is so important that you heal from this now and not have it hanging on for years to come."

Mentally on overload, I did not take in the full import of his words. But as the weeks wore on, it became clearer to me that I wasn't going to rebound in a flash. This was evidently going to be a long haul. Fortunately, the Baptistes remained at my side.

One afternoon, I ran into a bronzed and radiant Magaña returning from the beach. "Tomorrow," she announced excitedly, "we'll meet at the beach at 10:00 a.m. and take sand baths. They are so healing, Michele. They draw toxins out of the system, like a sauna. It will be a great experience for you, and you can do them regularly after we leave."

The next day the whole group of us arrived promptly at ten. Not feeling particularly well, I forced myself to leave the comfort of my hammock in hopes of feeling better. There in the sand, not too close to the water, were ten holes dug in a perfect row. They looked like burial plots. The sand was hot from the sun, but not yet burning. Magaña instructed us to climb in and lie down, and Miguel and Vicente used their shovels to bury us up to the neck, where we lay motionless with hats over our faces for sun protection. I felt the strange sensation of being gently compressed on all sides and baking slowly.

After twenty minutes or so, we sat up and ran into the ocean for a saltwater bath to wash off the thin layer of sand that completely covered our bodies. When I emerged from the water, I was amazed at how light I felt. Where before I was feeling heavy and sluggish, my movement through space was now effortless. I commented to Magaña about the noticeable difference.

"Yes," she nodded, "the forces of nature have great healing powers. Have you ever heard of putting clay on a bee sting to draw out the poison? Well, warm sand works much the same way. And it's been documented that ten minutes in salt water increases the oxygen level of the blood by two percent.

"Whenever I go into the ocean," she added, "I think of it as a cleansing ritual. Before entering, I ask the divine waters to purify me of any negativity whatsoever on any level—body, mind, or spirit. It's vital to remember always that the mind is so powerful, and the thoughts that you harbor will either contribute to your healing or detract from it."

Long before the inextricable connection between mind and body was accepted or even much known in the West, Walt and Magaña taught that we are beings with powers of self-healing far beyond what we know, and that by harnessing the powers of the mind and breath, we can initiate wellness in every aspect of our being.

"There's nothing new about this," Magaña said to me. "We all have an innate healing intelligence. Hippocrates said 'the natural healing force in each of us is the greatest force in getting well.'"

"But Magaña," I pleaded, "it's so hard to settle down and do these practices when I'm not feeling well. My mind is so caught up in how miserable I feel, and I forget."

She lovingly took my hand in hers. "You can access your healing intelligence at will. First, you must lie down several times during the day, breathe deeply, and simply relax. When you consciously release physical and mental tension and relax into your spiritual essence, you tap into cosmic energy and spiritual power from which all healing comes."

Walt's philosophy of healing was to "leave no stone unturned." He had arrived in El Salvador with an entire suitcase for me, filled with vitamins, cleansing herbs, and books about healing the liver. Along with positive affirmations and deep meditative techniques that directed mind, breath, and light energy into parts of the body in need of healing, he stressed the role of nutrition. Each morning, he personally brought me special blender drinks using blood builders like tomato juice made from crushed fresh tomatoes. He'd often bring a hard-boiled egg as well, because the type of protein it contained was far better for the liver than heavier meat protein. In meals he prepared for me, he frequently served me beets and beet greens. "Beet is excellent for the liver," he pronounced, "and a wonderful blood builder." I obediently and gratefully ate every bite.

Magaña brought along an array of crystals and gemstones and taught me to place them on particular chakras, or spiritual energy centers, to stimulate my deepest restorative energies.

"You know from our work together," she reminded me, "that you are composed of other bodies besides your physical body. If one of your energetic bodies is out of balance or weak, the physical body will reflect that state. The crystals will help to balance the chakra energies and help stimulate your healing process." She then gifted me with a yellow gold citrine crystal to balance my solar plexus chakra, which governs the liver and gallbladder area.

The Baptistes also employed a system of color healing. One morning, we covered clear, water-filled drinking glasses with plastic pieces of red gel paper and placed them outside to absorb the sun's rays through the red color. We then drank the water after it sat in the sun for awhile, so that we would take into ourselves the essence of the color red—a blood builder. We sometimes used yellow and gold gels, whose colors were helpful for liver purification, as well as green to soothe inflammation. All of these healing modalities are based on the premise that we are far more than flesh and bone: we are beings of light energy, vibrating at high frequencies that are affected by other high vibrational influences such as *prana*, color, sound, and the elements of nature.

For some people—and apparently I was one—hepatitis A takes a long time to resolve. Each week I felt stronger and stronger as I basked in the Baptistes' nurturing treatments. But four weeks after they'd arrived, I still was not back to my usual level of energy, and my appetite flagged. I knew Walt and Magaña had to leave again to attend to things in San Francisco, but I resolved to continue all of the treatments they'd so thoughtfully prescribed.

On the day of their departure I took a walk on the beach and stopped to watch Magaña doing yoga from a distance. She performed what seemed to be hundreds of continuous cobra *asanas*, her heart open to the sky and her mane of black hair streaming in the tropical breeze. I watched her in awe and marveled at her stamina. I was certainly going to take her advice in matters of health, for she was the picture of it. As she walked back from the edge of the surf she noticed me, stopped, and took my hands in hers. "You will feel better and better, Michele," she assured me. "Sometimes the body just gets sick, but you have to take the time to make it whole again so you can move beyond it into other realms." Then she smiled and added tantalizingly, "You will see how well you will feel when the pyramid is finished, and you will see where you can go with it—and without it."

CHAPTER 16

THE PYRAMID

"The body resembles a garment. Go, seek the one who wears it; don't kiss a piece of cloth."
— RUMI, "THE WORLD"

*I*t was Magaña's idea to build a pyramid on the retreat property. Born in El Salvador, she strongly identified with the Mayan culture, and had made many pilgrimages with Walt to pyramids and sacred sites around the world, including the famous El Salvador Olmecan pyramid, Tazumal.

There are numerous theories of the origins of the pre-Colombian pyramids that can be found throughout southern Mexico and Central America. Some theories attribute their construction to the survivors of Plato's sunken island of Atlantis; some posit a mysterious connection between the Mayan civilization and ancient Egypt.

Universally, pyramids are associated with spirituality and mysticism. Although sometimes considered burial sites, as in ancient Egypt, they also served as temples for the spirits to travel to other dimensions of the afterlife.

Many secret societies throughout history have quietly embraced the teaching that pyramids can be used for initiation into greater spiritual knowledge and mystical practices leading to other realms and planes. According to these teachings, pyramids may be considered departure gates for inner voyages, so to speak, where the spiritual traveler has the ability to return to his or her material existence after a transcendent sojourn.

Pyramids are also associated with renewal and with the healing of body, mind, and spirit. They are said to promote and restore well-being by capturing and channeling universal energy, which is properly aligned and magnified by their geometric form. Some who have studied pyramids have contended that flowers grow faster, that foods improve in taste, and that the bodies of dead animals resist decay for weeks when placed within a pyramid.

Naturally, there are skeptics. But if pyramid power is a delusion, it is a ubiquitous delusion that has pervaded disparate cultures since civilization's birth. In addition to being appropriated by Egyptians as sacred tombs and by Mayans for religious ceremonies, pyramids are referenced in the ancient Hindu Vedas. Turn over a U.S. dollar bill and you will see a pyramid, widely thought to be a Masonic symbol, its separated cap hovering above an all-seeing eye. To the spiritual aspirant, the eye symbolizes the third eye or sixth chakra, which, when opened, allows entry to other realms. It seems that humans have intuitively been drawn to pyramids for profound reasons that are as real as they are inexplicable.

Our retreat pyramid was architecturally designed and executed by Walt to combine elements of the Great Pyramid of Giza and El Salvador's Tazumal. But as always, Gurudev contributed his originality, invoking special principles that would enhance spiritual experience. He employed twenty carefully chosen Salvadoran workers, descendents of ancient pyramid builders no doubt, to carry out construction that took well over a year to complete. Throughout the process, no electric equipment or tools were used, so as not to despoil the energy field.

Walt began by digging a huge hole (about twenty feet deep) and filling it with boulders. "I want a powerful base," he'd explained. "One that will withstand earthquakes and sinking soil."

I was immediately reminded of Gurudev's recurring theme for us students: *From a sound base upward.* He always encouraged us to build our foundation in such a way that we would not be easily swayed by the vicissitudes of life as we progressed upward on the spiritual path.

Because our pyramid sat on the far side of the property, and because there was so much additional construction going on, it went largely unnoticed at first. In the initial phases, work stopped altogether whenever Walt returned to San Francisco, but resumed immediately upon his return. Toward the end, he allowed the project to continue in his absence—albeit with careful instructions for the construction supervisor.

During the construction process, Magaña imbedded in the structure various crystals meant to enhance the structure with their vibrational energies relating to the chakras, as well as various stones that she had gathered from sacred sites around the world, including the Temple of Karnak in Egypt. She placed one powerful crystal at the pyramid's peak.

Upon completion, the pyramid was twenty-five feet tall, with a first floor that housed numerous small meditation areas and a small second story just under the apex. The structure was made entirely of brick and had steps up the sides created by the ascending brickwork. The entrance was protected by a formidable wooden door that took great strength to open and, once closed, shut out all outer light and sound. At the very top of the structure a concrete opening, eight inches in diameter, allowed air to enter, and Walt placed a blue corrugated covering over the opening so that during the daylight hours, the shining sun created a perfect blue circle on the floor of the small room at the pyramid's apex.

As construction was completed in the late fall of 1978, and the finishing touches were being added to the pyramid, the excitement among the group of students who had arrived for the initiation built to a crescendo. Some were anxious, others curious, and some of us, including Norman and me, viewed it as yet another high-level opportunity for real spiritual experience offered to us by the guru. To say we were eager to experience meditation in this sacred structure was an understatement. On a bright December day, fifteen of us were initiated into the pyramid together with great dignity and pomp.

We arrived at the front of the pyramid at ten in the morning with our requested flashlights to find Walt and Magaña standing solemnly at the entrance. Norman passed out blindfolds and asked us to place them firmly over our eyes so that no outer light could shine through. We were individually led through the main door of the pyramid to specific meditation benches. I could hear some of the students being led up a stairway. I was also aware of sharing my bench with someone else, but I had no idea who it was. Then we heard the large entry door shut tightly after us.

Magaña began speaking. "Please remove your blindfolds," she instructed. As she spoke, her voice, low and clear, seemed to come from another plane. I took off my blindfold but it made little difference. The room was pitch black.

We began by chanting "Om" together several times and then Magaña began the invocation, taking on the role of high priestess.

"We invoke higher spiritual energies on all planes of being. We invoke the angelic kingdoms and legions of light beings on all planes."

She rang a Tibetan bell three times, and the sound reverberated in the chamber until I could feel its vibration in my spine. "We are a brotherhood and sisterhood of light and we offer ourselves to the highest reality and sacred light energy."

Gurudev spoke next, with great power and eloquence. "We are given this sacred pyramid for higher instruction into the great within. The doorway to the pyramid is a metaphor for the entrance to our own inner worlds."

I barely had time to digest the magnitude of his words before he went on.

"As physical beings, we are taught that there are nine openings in the body. But there is a secret tenth opening, a spiritual door that few are given to know of, located at the crown of the head. Through consciousness, with keenness of attention—needlepoint sharpness—we may find our way through this opening. The high goal of the yogi is to open this tenth door and achieve union with the supreme Godhead."

Walt had referred to this tenth door in his classes in San Francisco. "The ultimate goal of the yogi is to die a conscious death," he taught. "The purpose of meditation is to learn how to die before dying."

Norman had told me that yoga masters throughout the ages have chosen their moment of death, and some have called on their disciples to be present. They sit down together in meditation and, at the selected moment, the master's spirit leaves the body through the crown of the head. Leaving the body through this secret opening is considered in spiritual circles to be the ultimate and highest form of death.

After his invocation, Gurudev led us into a long and deep meditation and entrusted us with sacred spiritual instruction. When the teachings were completed and the meditation came to a close, he encouraged us to practice daily. "The pyramid will be open day and night for your personal use. During this retreat period, if you want to see real results that will be of great benefit to you, spend a minimum of two hours in the pyramid with your mind focused at the top of the head, as if you could look right up out of the top of the head into the universe above."

Two-hour sessions in the pyramid. My mind was reeling.

"It takes profound concentration and daily steady practice, but you all have the capacity to do it or you would not be here."

I was aware of beads of sweat all over my body. The intensity of the rituals and the energy within the pyramid itself was overwhelming, and I found myself anxious to leave so as to reconnect with some sense of normalcy. As if in response to my discomfort, Magaña rang the bell, again three times, and closed the ceremony, again invoking hierarchies of divine light beings.

After the initiation, everything seemed to return to normal on the surface, yet I was very aware of having been rearranged on a deep cellular level. *It's why I'm here*, I reminded myself. I knew that my anxiety was fear of the unknown and fear of change. One of Norman's great pearls of wisdom penetrated my thoughts: "A yogi learns to become comfortable within the discomfort." As it turned out, my reaction was mild compared to that of some.

A few of the students were seriously freaked out. "No way will I go in again without Gurudev being right there with me," one quaking soul confided to me later that afternoon. I, on the other hand, found this mysterious refuge a little scary but irresistibly intriguing. I was convinced that it would help me on

my determined journey toward enlightenment. No way was I
going to pass up this opportunity. I'd gotten this far, and for me
there was no turning back.

The second time I went to the pyramid was before daybreak on the day following the initiation. I went on my own.
I wanted to explore my new meditation space more carefully
and hoped that I would have solitude while the others slept. It
took all my strength to open the outer door. With some trepi-
dation, I shone my handheld flashlight into a narrow corridor.
Although Walt had walked us through the space the day before,
I felt disoriented now. I looked carefully around and spied yet
another door four feet ahead of me. I opened it and came
upon a passageway leading to an inner chamber. On either side
of this second passageway, before entering the main chamber,
were two more heavy wooden doors. I opened them one at
a time to discover they sealed two antechambers for private
meditation. The one on the left had a built-in concrete bench
that faced east; the one on the right had a bench that faced
west. As I examined this second chamber, I shone my flashlight
directly onto a surprised scorpion clinging to the brick wall.
I made a mental note to quietly let Gurudev know we had an
unwanted intruder.

The inner chamber itself was not large, but it was the biggest
room in the pyramid. A large seat, presumably for the teacher,
was in the center facing the doorway. Four small concrete meditation benches, each big enough for just one person, were situated to faced four different directions, taking advantage of the
energies of that particular direction. (I once queried Gurudev
about the distinctions between each direction's powers, but
his cryptic answer didn't really surprise me. "Many cultures
have systems that explain all of this, from Native Americans to

Tibetans to the Chinese. But I want you to discover for yourself what each direction gives to you.")

On the right side of the inner chamber was a steep, narrow, concrete staircase that led to the upper chamber, or eye of the pyramid—which, in esoteric teaching, correlates to the eye in meditation. During the day, one could sit in the center of the blue circle of light, but in this predawn hour the space was pitch black. This small chamber fit three meditators. It was not high enough to stand in (you had to stoop over to climb in), but it was large enough for one person to lie down in. As it turned out, people were very respectful if they knew the upper area was occupied and generally waited until it was empty before entering.

Once I'd acclimated myself to the entire layout, I felt much more settled and ready to focus. I decided to return downstairs and sat on the meditation bench in the small, east-facing chamber. I was less than a minute into my meditation, or so it seemed, when I heard a huge crash, as if a pair of orchestra cymbals had been clanged together full out. Incredibly, the sound seemed to be coming from inside of me. In San Francisco, Walt had taught us about internal sounds that arise in deep meditative states—flutes, gongs, bells, the motor sounds of the body, the buzzing of a million bees—but I had never expected anything like this. And I certainly had not gone very deep yet. It took me awhile to collect myself, but I did so and then continued with my practice. The sound did not recur, but it was a harbinger of things to come. Over the coming months, this tiny chamber would become for me a room of great transport to unique spiritual experiences.

As time went by, virtually everyone who experienced the pyramid agreed that some of their most powerful meditative experiences occurred within its walls. Among them, the student who at first exhibited the most fear and resistance came to be its staunchest supporter. But perhaps the one who had the most intense incident of all was Norman.

Norman was with us for the pyramid initiation, and he took to meditating in it as ardently as I did. He couldn't wait to get in there in the morning and often preceded me in beginning his prescribed two-hour stint of practice. One morning, I watched him enter the pyramid at about 6:00 a.m. I set off to do a number of chores, including feeding the birds and livestock and exercising Naranja, all of which took some time. When I got to the pyramid at about 8:00 a.m., I climbed to the second story, hoping to take advantage of the brilliant early morning light that would be steaming in, and saw Norman sitting within the blue light circle. I assumed he would be finishing soon, and I returned back down to my usual lower chamber. Two hours later, I climbed the stairs again and was surprised to see Norman still there. He certainly did not appear to have moved; in fact, he looked as motionless as a statue. I couldn't help but stare at him for a few moments, admiring the depth of his concentration. He was so still I could not even see him breathe.

I exited the pyramid and went about my day, but at lunchtime I still had not seen Norman emerge. I couldn't imagine he was still meditating, but maybe he was. I put it out of my mind until I finally saw him ambling toward me across the beach in the late afternoon.

"Where've you been?" I asked him.

"Collecting myself," he said, smiling.

"Collecting yourself?"

"Yes. I was meditating in the pyramid, and when I was done,

well, I left. I went outside, stopped to look at the cashew nut tree and the flower bed next to it. I started to head for the kitchen, but then I realized I couldn't go any further."

"Why not?"

"I left something behind. I left my body. It was still inside the pyramid. I had to go back and get it."

I was flabbergasted. Walt had often talked about the astral body, the ethereal counterpart of the physical body. The astral body is said to be an energetic duplication of the physical form it envelops, and is attached to the physical body at the navel by a silver cord. According to the mystics, the astral body, accompanied by the mind, is capable of travel—astral projection—while the corporeal self sleeps, or meditates.

Norman's astral adventure struck me as undeniably true. It explained his preternatural stillness when I observed him in the pyramid. I was thrilled that my friend and mentor had shared this, especially since yogis do not generally talk about their spiritual experiences with others unless to help someone else on the path.

Walt had expounded on this unwritten rule in one of my early classes with him, and another great yogi, Swami Veda Bharati of India, has said, "A word spoken is power lost." Norman also had touched on it, telling me, "It's such a gift to have inner experience that you want to keep the energy inward to incubate and build. If you send it out and give it away by talking about it, you weaken it and lessen the chances to have the experience again."

"Is it like not talking about something you are planning until it happens?" I'd asked Norman.

"Exactly. Other minds are powerful, and the attitude of the person you share an experience with can have influence. If you have questions about something you experience, it is always best to ask the teacher or someone else you are certain will understand.

"And," he'd added, "be sure that you're not speaking of it out of ego. That can get tricky."

I knew right away that Norman sharing his out-of-body experience was meaningful and was serving a purpose that I did not yet completely understand.

I was also relieved that he was able to retrieve his body without incident. Walt was always clear that we should not meditate in venues where the body would be in any danger if we vacated it temporarily—hence a longstanding prohibition against meditating too close to the ocean's edge.

I was filled with questions. "How did you get back inside your body?"

"I went back inside where it was sitting and just floated into it," he answered. "It was effortless."

"What was it like to be in two places at once?" The questions flew out of my mouth. "Was it amazing? Was it scary?"

But now Norman just smiled his inscrutable smile and replied, "I'm hungry." He made for the kitchen once more, this time taking his legs, arms, and grumbling stomach with him.

⌒

Although I did not experience what Norman did, my many hours of meditation in the pyramid no doubt had a profound impact on my being at every level. One consequence was the expedition of my long hepatitis recovery. According to Walt's instructions, I would often spend meditation time in the east-facing chamber making my mind one-pointed, focusing on whatever light I found inside and directing it into my liver. How the pyramid's structure aided this practice I never knew, but most everyone came to believe in its curative powers for whatever ailed them.

Over the course of the Christmas school break, when the pyramid was first in use, Walt and Magaña's son, Baron Baptiste, then fifteen, came to stay and, being scientifically minded, decided to stage an experiment. He placed a pair of dead batteries beneath the pyramid's apex, in the blue circle, for three days. When he retrieved them, they once again powered his transistor radio.

Between the pyramid's power and my adherence to Walt's dictum that I take it easy during the summer and fall that the pyramid was being finished—which I did by taking up "hammock duty" while Amigo gently swung me to and fro—I came to feel like my proverbial old self again. But of course, there are no old selves, only new selves, evolving every moment. And once more, new challenges waited on the horizon.

CHAPTER 17

TWO DEATHS

*"When you were born, you cried, and the world rejoiced.
Live your life in such a manner that when you die, the
world cries and you rejoice."*

—KABIR

*I*n the month or so after the pyramid debuted, most of my
fellow students departed to resume their lives back in San Francisco. Walt, too, went back to take up his role at the Center.
It was January 1979, and back in the "real world" there were
big goings-on. America and China established full diplomatic
relations, the Khmer Rouge met defeat in Cambodia, and the
Shah fled Iran. I was as unfazed by any of this as I was, for now,
by the increasing violence in parts of El Salvador. In my retreat
cocoon, I was alone again—and happily so.

I was spending hours each day doing *kriya* work and meditation, and I used the pyramid frequently. The combination of
practices was so intense that, at times, I felt I was catapulted
into another reality. Once again, trips into town became unsettling. The stimulation was hard to bear. And I could not make
sense of why there were so many soldiers lurking about. I knew
only that I didn't like the "vibe" they brought to La Libertad.

Though market days were a necessity, I tried to complete my town-based errands as quickly as possible.

Back at the retreat, I felt completely safe and secure. I was under the impression that nothing could alter my blissful mindset once I was back at our idyllic slice of beach. But I was wrong.

One early March day, I was eating lunch in the surf room when I looked down and saw a commotion on the adjacent property, the property that belonged to Miguel and Maria, the kind couple who occasionally gave me a ride into town. From the number of people running toward the group that was already clustered at the shoreline, I knew that whatever happened was serious. Instinctively, I wanted to see if I could help. I let my plate clatter to the floor and ran toward the swelling crowd. To my horror, there were two bodies at the center of that crowd. Maria and Miguel had been pulled from the water, drowned.

It is never easy to comprehend a tragedy, and this one was no exception. I am sure I stood staring at the bodies blankly for some moments before my brain even registered what my eyes assured me was true. Once the reality of the situation began to sink in, I denied it. *They can't possibly be dead*, I thought. *The natives don't even go into the water here at this time of year. They know how strong the undertow can be.* Miguel and Maria and I had even talked about this—*joked* about it. They told me they grew up so leery of this treacherous surf that, like many Salvadorans, they had barely learned how to swim.

Gradually, I began to make some sense of the anguished snippets of talk coming from the onlookers around me. *Children in the water . . . pulled out to sea . . . Maria tried . . . she tried . . . Miguel got the children . . . Gracias a Dios. But then, then . . .*

I now understood. Maria had tried to save her young son and daughter, who'd been playing at the ocean's edge and gotten dragged into the water by a giant wave. Not being a swimmer, Maria started to go under. Miguel was somehow able to rescue the children, but then drowned in a failed attempt to pull his wife from the deep. Others had tried to resuscitate them; some had carried the children—*the poor children*—up to the house and were caring for them. Now no one could do anything. No one could do anything.

I stood mute, trying to process it all. I could not take my eyes off the two lifeless bodies. It was the first time I had ever seen bodies uninhabited by their souls, and at first I tried to look at them in a detached way. It was clear that Miguel and Maria were gone. They had given up their earthly lives so their children could keep theirs. What were left were simply the empty shells they had inhabited. I looked in the direction of their young children and my heart ached for their huge loss. I did not even realize I was weeping until a woman came up beside me and put a hand on my shoulder.

I don't remember much about the rest of that day. The hours passed in a haze. Somehow I got back to the retreat and got through the night with Amigo by my side. As dogs do, he had a way of knowing I was hurting and was determined to stand by me. His presence was the only thing that helped. I have a vague memory of trying, without success, to calm myself with prayer and meditation.

I felt, on top of all my grief and shock, profoundly disappointed in myself. Shouldn't a yogi be better able to get ahold of herself? Shouldn't I be more dispassionate? What was death, according to the teachings? It is the ceasing of the breath that links the mind to a particular body. But *one still exists.* Between lives—for there will be another life, and another—we are, as the sages say, "waves of bliss in the ocean of the Universe."

Still, I wept. The depth of grief I was experiencing was new to me, and I questioned myself as a yogi in the face of falling to pieces so completely.

What happened to my yogic skills? Where was my yogic peace of mind? All I could think of was that I had to get to La Libertad and call Walt, which I set out to do early the next morning. I believe I felt he would impart some words of wisdom to me that would heal my grief and restore my equanimity. He might say, *Death is a habit of the body*, or *Death is a necessary stage*. And he would inevitably say it in such a way that it would affect me on the deepest of levels. Then I could stop crying at last.

But Walt said none of those things. After expressing great compassion for the terrible tragedy, he addressed my anguish.

"Michele," he said gently, "you mustn't be upset because you're grieving. It's natural to feel your feelings. You are a yogi, and you are also a human being with human feelings. Don't deny your humanity."

At last I felt some true consolation. It was unnecessary to tie up my energy with misplaced guilt. I knew I could now cry solely and purely for Miguel and Maria and their now-orphaned boy and girl.

A few weeks later, Walt and Magaña came down with a group of students, as they would a number of times for the remainder of the year. Along with these formal group retreats came schedules to which we were expected to adhere. In the morning, after individual sunrise meditation, we all met for a brisk beach walk. Each day, Walt taught a Raja Yoga class in the late morning and a *pranayama* (breathing) and meditation session an hour after dinner. Magaña led daily movement classes in the afternoon that always picked up my energy and gave me such joy. Another student who particularly loved Magaña's classes was Randy, a very sober and serious San Francisco doctor who would totally loosen up during her sessions, moving with abandon and childlike glee.

One morning during a tropical fruit buffet breakfast under the glorietta, I noticed Gurudev standing outside the kitchen door, looking our way. He caught my eye and asked me to come over and to bring Randy with me. Randy and I stood at attention as Walt spoke to each one of us. It was clear that the information he was providing to us individually was meant for both of us to hear. After a few pleasantries, he addressed Randy.

"Randy, you are a great doctor and a real credit to your profession. You are a healer and your job is to heal people."

Then he looked at me. "Michele, you are not to heal people. Your job is to teach people to heal themselves."

Randy and I motionlessly waited to see what was coming next. A long pause was followed by a delighted smile. "That's it, kids," said Walt. "Have a beautiful day."

During this particular trip, Gurudev concocted yet another new plan to enhance our paradise. One day, he returned from town with a pickup truck filled with plastic tubs, tubes, bags of gravel, and tiny plants. He beckoned to our *guardián*, Carlos, to follow him, and they disappeared toward the beachfront. All morning, sounds of hammering and muffled instructions could be heard coming from the area. I was immensely curious—and more than a little apprehensive, given my lack of rapport with plants—but it was clear to me that whatever the endeavor was, I had not been invited. When the time was right, it would be revealed.

In the afternoon, Walt, pleased and sweaty, invited me to the unveiling of my new project. He opened a low gate to the newly created area, a small space of fifteen feet by eight feet. Eight large, plastic tubs filled with gravel had been placed upon a raised wooden platform. Sitting in the gravel were tiny vegetable plantings: tomatoes, bell pepper, cucumber, yellow squash, and green beans.

"This is your hydroponic garden," he proudly announced.

I hadn't a clue what a hydroponic garden was, but clearly it held a great measure of importance to the guru, so that was enough for me. He looked at me sharply and elaborated. In a standard garden, the plant received its nutrients from the soil and water. The difficulty with my previous gardening attempts, he said, was that both the soil and the water contained too much salt, being so close to the ocean. Although vegetable plants would grow to a certain point, they would not bear fruit. And although I had really tried on previous occasions, it was to no avail.

And so I had a gardening reprieve. And many new instructions to follow.

"Because these plants are in gravel and not soil," Walt explained, "they must be fed nutrients three times a day at regular intervals—early morning, noon, and late afternoon, with this special mixture that you will add to water." I was to pour the mixture into a large tub that had tubes leading from it to the seven smaller plastic tubs. When the smaller tubs filled, the water was to sit in them for fifteen minutes, then be drained through small openings in the bottoms.

Before Walt left at the end of that trip, he gave me another practice to do in his absence. This particular *kriya* practice was to be done one hour in the morning, one hour at noon, and one hour in the late afternoon. "Use a clock," he said. "The one hour is not to count for other practices, only this practice."

It suddenly dawned on me that the hydroponic garden and the *kriya* breath were two related practices. I was, in effect, watering my chakras, providing spiritual *kundalini* nutrition to my chakra system. Once again, I realized that the guru was giving me a deeper teaching through the garden project that was to give me more insight into his metaphorical instruction on the waters of life.

Once I was alone again, I faithfully worked on perfecting the new practice Walt had taught me. Doing such intense *kriya* work for several hours a day, I knew, could help one achieve purification on many levels. I wanted to make my mind an appropriate vessel for the spiritual forces that might infuse it. In short, I wanted to be ready for enlightenment, should it be ready for me. Older and wiser than I was when I began my quest, I knew by now that one could not call in an order for enlightenment and have it delivered. But one must be ready for it when it comes. So I strove for the clarity of mind that is a necessary precondition for enlightenment, and that was easiest to do in silence and solitude, without—as they said in the *Star Wars* movie I had finally seen during my last stint in San Francisco—any "disturbance in the Force."

Whenever I was by myself, the entire retreat became my temple. I was drawn deeper and deeper into an ethereal realm. But as a consequence, I sometimes was less conscious of my physical surroundings than I might have been otherwise. One night, walking in the dark without a flashlight, I tripped over a slumbering Amigo and jammed the middle toe of my right foot into a door. I instantly knew the toe was broken. Any doctor will tell you there is "nothing you can do" for a broken toe, and I hobbled around on it for a few weeks without it seeming to get much better.

Fortunately for me, Norman arrived at the retreat. Learning of my plight, he went to his room and emerged with a batch of French green clay, one of many natural remedies in his traveling medicine chest. He mixed the green powdery substance with water in a clay bowl and stirred it with a stick—"No metals," he warned me—until it formed a paste, which he applied liberally to my crushed and swollen digit. In the end, my foot healed much more quickly than it normally would have. And, to my amazement, in three days I was no longer hobbling. In fact, my balance was so well restored that Baron, again visiting during a school break, was able to teach me to surf.

Surfing was great fun and became a passion for me. It seemed a fitting way to round out inner balance with outer balance. Nevertheless, I was always cognizant of the ocean's power, and determined to be respectful of it. I had not forgotten the lesson of Maria and Miguel.

And so this year, yet another year in a world so different from that of my contemporaries, rapidly drew toward its close. I had not been back to the States at all in 1978 or 1979, and had no particular desire to go. I was content dividing my time between weeks of contemplative solitude and weeks of socializing as I helped to acclimate our visitors. When Walt, Norman, and Baron arrived in early December, ahead of a larger group who were scheduled to stay through Christmastime, I was about ready for some camaraderie and looked forward to the festivities.

Soon after the three of them settled in, we had our first celebration: Baron Baptiste's sixteenth birthday party. Walt had cooked Baron's favorite dinner, Hawaiian-style prawns with pineapple, tomatoes, and a touch of curry, and the meal was to be served in the surf room. Norman, Baron, and I were upstairs sitting at the dinner table enjoying the aftermath of a magnificent sunset, when we realized the lights didn't work. Soon it would be dark. Upon closer inspection, it became evident that some of the electrical wires had become corroded with salt. They were completely frayed. I ran downstairs and brought some candles, but the wind was so strong they would not stay lit. It looked like we would have to change our venue. Then Walt ascended the stairs, carrying an enormous platter of shrimp.

"What happened to the lights?" he asked.

But before I could finish my explanation, the electricity kicked in. The room was totally illuminated. I heard Baron say under his breath, "Thanks, Dad."

They say that *guru* means "one who brings us from darkness to light." In this case, the definition was literal. As I had many times before, I marveled at the extent of Walt's abilities and wondered about their limitations. But, I was soon to be reminded that there were certain events that had to play out for reasons of karma.

About a week later, a number of additional students arrived. A large group of us were sharing a communal dinner outdoors when it occurred to me that someone was missing. I had not seen Amigo in awhile. In itself, this was not so unusual. Amigo would sometimes disappear for an entire day, taking off over the wall by the *estero* and exploring the jungle. But he had an uncanny way of arriving home for dinner when our guests were numerous, sensing that if he lurked around long enough someone would slip him some tasty scraps. Yet, this night Amigo did not come back.

The following morning, I awoke to the news that Amigo was back, and sick. I raced down to see him and found Walt tending to him.

"He jumped back over the wall, Michele," Walt said. "But he's not well."

At that very moment, Amigo began to have a convulsion. He was thrashing around and foaming at the mouth. At the same time, you could see that Amigo was trying desperately not to hurt anyone. It was so awful to watch that I had to turn away. This was unthinkable! Walt had to do something!

"He may have been bitten," Walt said, "or he may have eaten a poisonous snake."

Carlos tried to hold Amigo while Walt poured a liquid down the dog's throat. "What's that?" I asked. "What are you giving him?"

"I'm trying to get a big dose of vitamin C in him, to counteract the poison," Walt said. But something about his voice told me this was far from a sure cure.

Hours went by while we tried to get Amigo to drink some water and waited to see if the vitamin C would have any impact. Nothing seemed to help. Ultimately, Amigo went completely out of control and had to be put inside the gym to ensure he would not hurt himself or anyone else. I was crying hysterically, and begged Walt to take him to a hospital in La Libertad. But, as Walt tried to explain to me, Amigo would be impossible to transport—and this remote part of El Salvador was not the sort of place you could rush a dog to an animal hospital. Here, wild dogs roamed freely. Here, even humans had a hard time getting medical attention.

I knew Walt would have done something, anything, within his power to save Amigo, for the two of them shared a bond that was stronger even than my own. But we all knew what was going to happen, and, later that night, it did. My dear Amigo was gone.

In the face of this death, I needed no one's permission to experience the full depth of my grief. I sobbed and wailed until I had no more tears to spill and no voice left with which to ask, "Why?" Walt let me do what I had to do, and as with Miguel and Maria, did not try to soothe me with homilies. He just let me be.

I knew I was going to be profoundly sad for some time, and that was just the way it had to be. But once my tears were spent, I did take some comfort in what I knew from the teachings. Certain animals, they say, are more evolved than certain people. A noble beast like Amigo was very likely destined to come back in human form, where he could continue to further his own spiritual growth. I held that wish for the dog that had been my loving companion. And few things seemed more certain to me than that our paths will cross again. But in the meantime, I knew things would be different for me here without my best friend.

CHAPTER 18

A MEETING WITH MY BROTHER

*"After your mother has given birth to you, and your par-
ents have raised you, then the role of the guru begins, and
he helps you fulfill the purpose of your life."*

—SWAMI RAMA

*I*n 1980, the political situation in El Salvador was heating up.
Fortunately, La Libertad was spared much of the upheaval, in
part because of the presence of the Salvadoran Navy, whose
small base was located near the pier. In addition, the isolation of
our retreat, outside of town, two miles from the highway with
only a one-road access, provided a buffer from the violence
erupting throughout the nation.

In early January, Kate, who had returned to El Salvador for
the Christmas retreat, took a taxi into La Libertad to call her
parents and let them know her arrival date and time of her
flight home. Because she had spent some months at the retreat
earlier, she felt confident going into town alone, and the taxi
driver agreed to wait for her at the phone company.

When she got back to the retreat a few hours later, she took
me aside.

"I got stopped coming back," she told me, her eyes wide.

"Stopped? What do you mean? Who stopped you?"

"By a truckload of soldiers. They pulled my taxi over to the side of the road between here and Libertad, took my passport and the driver's, and ordered us to stay in the car. They kept our passports for a very long time, and all the armed soldiers in the back of the open truck kept staring at us. I'm not sure exactly how long but it seemed like an eternity. I was really scared, Michele. And I could tell the taxi driver was frightened, too.

"I couldn't think what to do so I just began mentally repeating my mantra. As soon as I started saying it quietly to myself, the door of the truck opened and two soldiers came over, handed us our passports, and motioned for us to leave."

She paused for a moment.

"Thank God for that mantra," she said. "It totally shifted the energy."

Kate's story was confounding to me. What could it mean? Why stop a young woman alone in a taxi? "Have you told Gurudev and Magaña?" I asked.

"Yes," she answered. "I told them as soon as I got back."

Kate and the rest of her group left the next day, although Walt and Magaña stayed on another week to take care of business in the capital city of San Salvador. When we were alone, Gurudev took me aside and reminded me to always carry my passport with me and to keep my shopping trips into La Libertad short. "Don't get personal with people in town," he cautioned me, "and you will be fine."

I took his advice to heart, but otherwise put the matter out of my mind.

After the Baptistes' departure, I spent the next three months in blissful solitude once more, with plenty of time for my spiritual practice, the hydroponic garden, surfing, and riding the horses. Enjoying my relaxed routine in the bosom of the retreat's beauty and serenity, I was completely content to be alone in harmony with the natural richness of life surrounding me.

The only wrinkle was the occasional worried look I would catch on our *guardián* Carlos's face when he listened to the radio. It was obvious the news was not good, and although he would sometimes try to fill me in on the country's turmoil, most of the details were beyond my Spanish vocabulary. I knew enough to surmise that there were real problems in the capital with a rising guerilla faction and violence between the guerillas and the army. One day, though, Carlos seemed unusually upset and made a real effort to communicate, trying several different methods to get me to understand. I picked up that someone important, a *padre*—a priest—named Romero had been killed. But the name meant nothing to me at the time. Finally, Carlos became exasperated by our language barrier and went back to his chores.

April in El Salvador is typically a month where the weather becomes unbearably hot and sticky. The humidity continues to build until May, when the rainy season begins to cool things off and provide a measure of relief. This year, the heat and humidity were the worst I had ever experienced, and during the night I would awaken two or three times to find myself covered in sweat. Half asleep, I would cool off with a cold shower before dropping back into a deep slumber. I was thankful to be living on the ocean and not in town, where after 10:00 a.m. it was difficult to function.

After five months without rain, the gardens, although watered regularly by Vicente and Carlos, were starting to show signs of distress, so I decided to supplement Vicente's watering with an extra shift of my own.

As I watered the thirsty bougainvillea, my thoughts turned to my imminent return to the U.S. It had now been almost two and a half years since my last trip home. During Walt's previous visit, we had talked about my leaving.

"These last two years have been important for you, Michele. I'm so thankful that you are strong and well. You have done very well for yourself and it shows in many ways. But it's time for you to return to San Francisco. You are needed there and they are waiting for you."

Two and a half years! It was incredible that so much time had elapsed. I had no regrets, but neither did I feel any resistance to returning. In fact, unlike the last time I departed El Salvador, I was genuinely excited. For much of the time I'd been here during this most recent stint, I had been well aware that my health was not up to city life, and that working would have been out of the question. Rest was what I needed and the retreat was the perfect environment. Now, I was ready. There is a season and cycle for everything, and a new cycle was on the horizon. Once again, the timing was perfect.

"I'd like to have a break in between and go back to Cleveland to visit my family," I told Walt.

"Absolutely," he agreed. "Why don't you take a month? I'll be coming back in May with a group of students. One of them will be Janice, my personal assistant. She can take over as manager. You can plan on leaving a few days after we arrive."

Walt's suggestion about spending a month in Cleveland had gotten me thinking about old times. So, on this steamy morning, as I continued to water the garden, I smiled to myself, thinking of how nice it would be to see my family again. But my thoughts were interrupted by Vicente, who was hurrying toward me.

"*Señorita Michele*," he called out.

"*Sí, Vicente?*" I replied, as I turned off the water and set the hose down.

"*Tu hermano está aquí,*" he said excitedly.

Ah, the language barrier again. I was sure I had misunderstood. It sounded like he'd said my brother was here. But that was ridiculous. I mentally ran through the list of my five brothers, but could not imagine any of them here in El Salvador. It had to be a mistake. Nevertheless, from Vicente's gesturing, I was pretty sure that someone or other was *aquí*, and I quickly ran to the front gate. There, in flesh and blood, stood my brother Martin, grinning from ear to ear.

"Hello, Michele," he said matter-of-factly, clearly amused at the stunned expression on my face. I regained my composure and threw my arms around him.

"Marty, Marty, what in the world are you doing here?" I asked with a mixture of shock and delight.

But his reply stunned me.

"I've come to take you back to America," Martin answered firmly. "Mom and Dad are very concerned about you and want you to come back now."

Of all of my five brothers, Martin held a very special place in my heart. He was the middle boy, seven years my junior, and had the most even temperament imaginable.

When I was nine and he was two, I wrote a play about us, entitled *The Day Marty and I Went to Florida*, which I cast, produced, directed, and starred in, presenting it for my fourth grade class. Although sibling arguments are a natural part of family life, and there were plenty of them in my family, Martin and I never clashed. I loved and trusted his goodness completely.

"How long can you stay?" I asked.

"I only have four days," he replied. "And in that time I intend to convince you to come back."

I decided to ignore his dictum for now and focused on getting my brother settled in the kitchen, where I made him coffee and breakfast. I was confident that once he was a bit rested I could talk some sense into him. But he continued to harp on how I had to leave *right away*.

"Look, Marty," I said, firmly digging in my heels, "I have one month left here and then I'm going back to Cleveland to visit the folks for a month. I can't leave the retreat now with no one here. I have a duty, and it's my responsibility to see it out to the end. There is no way I am leaving early."

Judging by the expression on his face, I could see he was not convinced, and we both decided to shift the conversation for the time being.

I held out my hand. "Come, let me show you around paradise."

Martin was a big teddy bear of a man, six foot two, with sparkling blue eyes and shaggy, light brown hair. He had followed in our father's footsteps, taking up the oboe at an early age and studying for years with John Mack, the first oboe of the Cleveland Orchestra. My brother was a talented musician who, even at his tender age, had played with some of the great orchestras in the world. He was playing with the Mexico City Symphony and had just returned from the orchestra's tour of Japan.

As it turned out, it was great to have his companionship, and for the next few days—just as when we were children—we played to our hearts' content. We rode down the beach to Playa de San Diego on the horses, where I introduced him to a few of the young men who worked at the retreat. Almost everyone commented on Marty's Spanish and wanted to know why his accent was so good and mine so bad. He couldn't *possibly* be my brother with such good Spanish, they joked. "I live in Mexico," he explained. Still, they shook their heads in awe. Perhaps they were wondering if I'd been adopted.

Marty and I swam in the ocean, floated in the pool, took long walks, ate delicious meals, and used the meditation room together. By the third day of his visit, he looked relaxed and happy, and I let myself believe that any worry for my safety seemed to have disappeared in the face of my healthy and happy regime.

Martin had always had a strong spiritual inclination and had experienced a meditation class with Walt during one of his visits to San Francisco. He seemed impressed at the time, and we had a lively conversation about perception and altered states of consciousness. I assumed that he was aware of the depth of my devotion to my spiritual development and the reasons for my service to my teacher. It had become so natural to me, so much a part of my reality, that I didn't fully consider how the outside world might interpret my unorthodox choice of lifestyle.

Three days into his visit, as we were sitting in the shelter of the courtyard sipping on coco water, Marty broached the subject of my homecoming again. What I hadn't realized was that Marty had heard a great deal from my mother and father about their extreme upset with my long absence, coupled with concern for my health and safety. Their concern had grown deeper ever since a man named Jim Jones, leader of something called Peoples Temple, persuaded more than nine hundred of his followers, Americans living in Jonestown, Guyana, to commit suicide by drinking a cyanide-laced grape drink. The media attention raised deeply unsettling questions in my parents' minds that continued to fester as stories on cult behavior and "deprogramming" proliferated.

"Look, Michele," Marty said, "Dad and Mom are really unnerved. They're worried about you—that Jim Jones thing, the hepatitis, the politics down here. You've been in El Salvador for a very long time and the situation is unraveling every day. You clearly have no idea how many soldiers with machine guns are in the airport and on the roads. When the archbishop was murdered, that was the last straw."

I pricked up my ears. "What archbishop?" I asked.

"Oh my god," he said with astonishment. "You don't know? It's all over the news. Archbishop Romero, the head of the Catholic Church here, was murdered in San Salvador last month while saying Mass, shot through the heart. He was a strong advocate for the poor and was against U.S. aid to the government. All hell is about to break loose."

A light bulb went off in my head. Finally, I understood what Carlos had been trying to tell me. I didn't know the word for "archbishop" so he had used the word for priest.

Marty hesitated briefly, then went on. "The folks are worried that maybe you've been brainwashed."

I sighed inwardly, resigned to the fact that the core of my spiritual belief system and my allegiance to my guru was about to be questioned by someone who I had thought supported me.

"Marty, right now, at this time of my life, I'm an apprentice. Think back to when you started studying the oboe. Dad made sure that you studied with one of the best oboe teachers in the world. You didn't just study with him for a year or two. It wasn't casual. You studied diligently, day after day, for many years, so he could pass his knowledge and experience on to you and guide you in the subtleties of the instrument."

"Yes," he countered, "but my teacher didn't dictate my whole life. I could still make my own decisions outside of music. This has taken over your entire existence."

"I can only tell you that what I am being given back is far, far more than I've given. I've always had the freedom of choice. One of the signs of a real spiritual teacher is that the student is free to go at any time. Walt has always said that he doesn't want weak followers who believe blindly. He wants students who have firsthand experience of what he is teaching. And I have been given experience that has shown me there is much more to life than the world teaches us."

"But what about this whole guru thing?" Marty persisted. "There are plenty of spiritual people out there who say you don't need a guru. That you can attain enlightenment on your own."

I had heard that argument before. I paused for a moment to find the right words. "Think of Mozart, Marty. He wrote his first symphony at the age of five and the original manuscript had no changes. But how many Mozarts are there? It's my understanding that throughout history there have been a few advanced souls who have been able to finally achieve enlightenment on their own, but it's very rare. Ego is tricky, Marty. There are deep recesses of the subconscious mind that must be conquered, as well as inner worlds. Most souls who are ready for the journey need a guide to show them the way, and I'm one of those souls who need that.

"That's what I'm doing here, studying with Walt Baptiste. The purposeful evolution of consciousness is a huge undertaking. When a spiritual student comes as far as he can go in a particular dimension of consciousness, the spiritual master guides the soul through to the next level. A spiritual master is someone who was at one time like us, and has gone on to do what it takes to attain God realization, or enlightenment. It's a guru's job to guide other souls on the path. He's already traversed the pitfalls and tricks of the ego, so he understands clearly what the disciple needs to do next to move to the next stage of consciousness."

Martin silently contemplated my words as I went on.

"It's said that when the time is right, God sends the perfect teacher for you. When the student is ready, the teacher appears. Walt has never asked me to leave the world. In fact, he wants his students to be successful in the material world. You've been to the Center in San Francisco, and you've seen for yourself how balanced the teachings are. Sure. I'm down here now for a few years of my life, but it's only to go back to the world stronger than I was when I left it."

I paused for a moment as Marty's expression softened.

"Marty," I implored, "you can see for yourself that I'm not in danger here. Things may be going on in other parts of the country, but not in this area. And besides, I'm careful. I know how to get around unobtrusively, and I don't go to the capital. I'm going back to the States in one month and I'm not about to leave my spiritual post until then."

He gently responded, "Where are you going with all this, Michele? Do you see yourself working for the Baptistes for the rest of your life?"

"No," I said.

"Well, what do you envision for your future?"

Without hesitation I replied, "I see myself teaching yoga."

It was interesting to me how fast those words sprung from my lips. During Walt's last visit, I had been clearing dishes when I overheard him say to some others still seated at the dinner table that he thought I would go on to be "an outstanding yoga teacher." I was so overwhelmed that I nearly dropped my stack of plates. I am not sure what startled me more, the fact that Gurudev had a vision of my future, or the reality that, sooner or later, there would be a future for me that was far more independent of this place, of the Center, and even of Walt.

CHAPTER 19

MY RED CARPET YEAR

"When you are in harmony, life becomes like a red carpet that rolls out before you."

—WALT BAPTISTE

*I*n spite of Marty's attempt to "rescue" me, I remained in El Salvador for a month after his visit until Walt and Magaña's arrival with a group of students. I saw Walt only briefly as he was being helped upstairs to his house. "Gurudev's not feeling well," Magaña explained.

During my first visit to El Salvador, Walt had shared with me that he suffered occasional recurring malaria symptoms from a bout with the illness that he picked up on a trip to India years before. That was the only time he ever referred to it, and although a few times over the years I could see in his eyes that he was not well, he never complained and went about his work inspiring everyone around him. Because he had told me this in confidence, I never said a word to anyone. I assumed the malaria had kicked in again. I had four days remaining before my plane would take me back to the States, and during the entire time Walt remained in his quarters.

By now I had learned that to worry about a guru is a misplaced sentiment.

There is karma in everything, and some spiritual teachings say that often when a guru is ill it is because he is taking on the karma of a student—lessening its effect on a situation that must be played out.

Walt always emphasized the importance of using the mind in healing. "When someone you love is sick, the best thing you can do is to envision the loved one surrounded in light. Every time you think of that person, see her surrounded by divine light." It made such beautiful sense. The mind is so powerful. If we visualize a person ill and infirm, we are sending out those negative thought waves. Better to use our minds as divine healing agents for those we love. And so I did.

The morning of my departure, Magaña, looking serene and confident, came to me with a message. "Gurudev is doing much better, Michele, but he's still resting. He asked me to wish you well on your journey and to have a wonderful time with your family. We love you dearly and look forward to seeing you in San Francisco."

⌒

The journey to Cleveland was a blur. One moment I was saying good-bye to my beloved ocean in the wilds of Central America, and the next moment I was hugging my parents in the parking lot of the Cleveland airport. What amazed me is that it seemed so perfectly natural, as though one event were designed to follow the other—another example that there is a divine order in the larger scheme of things.

My parents were beyond thrilled to see me and to observe

that I was still the Michele they knew. My father gave me a big hug and my mother was visibly relieved to have me home safe and sound, looking healthy and well. In fact, I was sporting a golden tan and was filled with energy despite the air travel. Nevertheless, my mother and father remained very concerned about my health in the wake of my hepatitis episode.

Through a family friend's connection, I quickly got an appointment with a top liver specialist at the renowned Cleveland Clinic where, after a battery of tests, I was given a completely clean bill of health. Now that my liver, like my personality, had been judged perfectly normal, relief was evident all the way around.

As it turned out, my visit to Cleveland yielded another happy result. Through a friend, I met a warm-hearted, fun, and good-looking man named Rob—a very successful entrepreneur, and somewhat older than I. He was completely different than anyone I had previously been attracted to—very strong and self-assured, yet a bit fragile from a recent divorce. He was fascinated by my El Salvador saga and taken with my fresh-off-the-retreat innocence. We hit it off, and spent a good deal of time together.

I alternated between time with my family and a whirlwind romance with him. This seemed to sit well enough with my parents, until the night I didn't come home. When I phoned them in the morning to let them know I was okay, my mother's icy "thank you for calling" could have frozen the equator.

An old defiance crept into me. *I'm thirty-two years old*, I thought. *I've been by myself for a long time. This wonderful man has come into my life, and I am going for it.* Much later, I came to acknowledge that in returning to Cleveland, some old patterns and deeper needs were still playing themselves out. As much as I had changed in so many ways, there were parts of the "old" Michele surfacing that I had not seen in a long time. I had never felt complete without a boyfriend in tow. This had been a source of continual friction between my parents and me throughout my young adult years.

"Living in the world is tricky," Norman had once said. "And going back to your roots can open up parts of yourself that are deeply imbedded in the psyche. That is why so many monasteries in the East have rules that require the aspirant to change his name and give up his family."

Yet, Walt had always encouraged us to live life to its fullest while remembering who we really were in our essence. I gratefully acknowledged my current exciting life chapter as a gift and an opportunity to experience the world as it was unfolding before me here in Cleveland. To stay as aware and grounded as possible, I kept up my meditation practice throughout, albeit a shorter version.

To my mother's credit, she recovered more quickly than I would have thought possible, and was even encouraging when Rob invited me to accompany him on a trip to New York City. I agreed to accompany him, excitedly thinking what a contrast it would be to visit the Big Apple after my years in rural Central America. I had no idea!

Rob was evidently even more well-heeled than I had realized. We flew first class, and stayed in his company-owned penthouse of a chic hotel, where the concierge fell all over himself trying to anticipate Rob's and my every need. One night we went to dinner at the legendary 21 Club and, just like in the movies, someone at a nearby table sent over a bottle of Dom Pérignon. Even in 1980, that gesture must have cost hundreds of dollars. Did people really live like this? Apparently they did. As we continued to do the town—wining, dining, shopping, and even making a foray to New Jersey's Monmouth Park Racetrack, where we sat in box seats on a glorious May afternoon—I truly felt like a fairy princess.

Then the clock struck twelve and my cosmopolitan week came to an end. After a final week in Cleveland, I bade good-bye to my family again and returned to San Francisco. I felt a bit deflated on the plane ride out, remembering the last time I'd headed to Northern California for a gloomy, gray June. I wondered if I'd be working in the restaurant again and living in my old room at the Center. One thing I should have learned by now was that, as they say, you never step into the same river twice. As usual, the San Francisco skies were gray as spring rolled into summer. But my time here was to be a sunny interlude, in part thanks to another new friend.

Taking up my post at the Hungry Mouth again, I ran into a new waiter, Horacio, a tall, dark, and handsome Colombian. Horacio told me in his distinctively low and sexy voice that he was one of the principal dancers with the San Francisco Ballet. He had, he said, fallen in love with Walt and the teachings and was working part-time in the restaurant as a form of Karma Yoga—service to the guru.

On hearing I needed a place to live, Horacio offered to get me into his building, an apartment complex nicknamed Heart-break Hotel in deference to its history as a brothel. I managed to lease a small studio apartment there, which suited me perfectly, as it was right across the street from the ocean with a direct view of the sea. The proximity to the water allowed me to somewhat reconnect with my Salvadoran beach. It also allowed me to keep up my surfing.

With Horacio's eager assistance, I had the time of my life decorating my tiny new space, but it never achieved the exotic flavor of Horacio's much larger apartment, which was decked to the ceilings with colorful art, flowing scarves, and large silk swatches. Always flamboyant, Horacio kept me laughing and on the go. Always elegant, sometimes improbably so, he met me several times a week for a run through Golden Gate Park, for which he invariably wore a gorgeous royal-blue cashmere sweater.

My friendship with Horacio was a highlight in my life. Sometimes we would talk for hours about Walt's spiritual teachings and the impact he was having on our lives. At other times, we would simply hang out and entertain each other with our unfolding life adventures. He was a true spiritual brother, and he gave me the gift of firsthand experience with the professional ballet world. He made sure that I often received premier tickets to the San Francisco Ballet, and on a few occasions got me backstage to view performances. I would miss Horacio terribly whenever he left town to tour with the ballet, but I consoled myself by house-sitting for him, feeding his fish and attempting to soak up a bit of his innate glamour by osmosis.

For a full year I lived on the ocean, surfed, and worked at the Center. After awhile I began working less in the restaurant and more upstairs at the yoga studio, where I assumed Janice's old post at the yoga center desk while she remained in El Salvador. I continued, too, to rotate through the boutique and the health food store, learning all aspects of the businesses and availing myself of large and welcome doses of Magaña and Norman.

As always, I remained devoted to the gym and began coaching others, including San Francisco Ballet dancers drawn to the Center by Horacio. I learned from both Walt and Norman how to design gym programs depending on the needs and desires of the individual. Many times Walt, upon request, would design a program and have me teach it to the student. This was a huge education for me, as the exercise programs addressed a variety of therapeutic needs (back issues, breathing problems, obesity), while also serving those who wanted intensive bodybuilding programs. Of course, there were also my own workouts designed by Walt, which I executed to the letter.

Rob, my sophisticated friend from Cleveland, came to visit me a few times that year, but at the end of his second weekend visit he broke the news.

"Michele," he said, taking my hand over a candlelight dinner in an elegant restaurant, "you are a great lady, but I can't relate to your lifestyle. I think we should go our separate ways. Yoga is more important to you than I am." Although I thought I took it pretty well, two days later I broke down and wept. I had opened my heart and now it was broken. What was wrong with me? Would I ever find a soul mate?

Walt had a class that evening, and although I was scheduled to work the front desk, Norman took one look at me and suggested I take the class instead while he covered for me.

Once again, Gurudev hit the nail on the head. As if speaking directly to me, he began the class talking about love. "God is perfect, ever-flowing love. Human love can fail you, but God love is forever, everlasting and dependable no matter what. To know God's love is to become within yourself the greater and better lover, not just of a personal nature but capable of a broader and more expansive, all-encompassing love for more of life and its manifestations and beings."

"Love God before and above all else," he said, "and you will be a better person. You will be happier in your existence, and you will become acquainted with life's higher meanings. Don't worry so much about being loved. Instead, be more of what love is."

After my relationship with Rob ended, the bulk of my social life was devoted to the many friends in our thriving spiritual community. A new level of camaraderie and joy settled into the yoga center. We were all growing, life was full, and at last I felt truly at home. There were times when I thought of El Salvador, to be sure. As content as I was and as devoted, as always, to my yoga and meditation, I knew I would never be able to practice here with the same intensity I could in that enchanted place. Despite the political mayhem now raging in many parts of that country, I still thought of it as a spiritual oasis. That is why I was devastated, in December of 1980, to pick up a newspaper and learn that three American nuns, Maura Clarke, Ita Ford, and Dorothy Kazel, along with a church worker, Jean Donovan, had been abducted, raped, and shot to death in El Salvador. Their bodies were found on the outskirts of La Libertad. Evidently, they were suspected of sympathizing with the leftist insurgents. My parents were beside themselves, especially since one of the women was from Cleveland. To make matters worse, a few months previous to the murders, my mother had received a phone call from her parish priest, who said he had heard they had a daughter in La Libertad, and if she ever needed help, she should contact these very nuns.

After the nuns were murdered, Walt had everyone at the retreat return to San Francisco, leaving the property in the care of the *guardiáns*. Although the event was prominent in the San Francisco papers, it soon died down as other world events like the Iran hostage crisis and the upcoming presidential election took center stage. El Salvador was no longer front-page news.

After several uneventful months had passed, Walt and Magaña

returned to El Salvador to see and feel out the situation for themselves. They found La Libertad to be safe and our secluded area to be untouched. Upon their return, Walt again asked me if I would like to go back for a while. "It's completely your decision, Michele. But it is there for you if you choose it."

The very next day, while on duty at the Hungry Mouth, I waited on a customer who turned out to be a Salvadoran living in San Francisco. The young man told me he was going down soon to visit an uncle who owned a farm in the center of the country. One thing led to another, and I found myself giving him directions to the retreat and invited him to visit if he was in the vicinity. There had to be some karmic message in it all, I surmised, for this young man to show up at our restaurant.

Now I knew my decision was made. For all the fun I was having, I longed for the blessed environment that could, I knew, take my practice to its highest levels. I wanted to continue my quest full out, just one more time.

CHAPTER 20

LOVE, FEAR, AND FAREWELL

"And the end of all our exploring will be to arrive where
we started and know the place for the first time."
—T.S. ELIOT

*I*n the spring of 1981, I returned to El Salvador. This time, the
soldiers at the San Salvador airport formed a thick swarm. The
feeling of foreboding that hung in the air was oppressive. It hung
heavier than the humidity, weighing everyone and everything
down. But I simply assumed that things would be lighter and
brighter when I reached my beloved retreat.

In a way, my expectations were met. The setting itself was as
peaceful and beautiful as ever. The coco trees, the pristine beach,
the crashing waves were all so exquisitely familiar and comforting
that I wanted to weep with joy. In a moment of abandon, I glee-
fully kicked off what I had come to think of as my "San Francisco
shoes" and wriggled my toes in the sand. It gave me such pleasure
to realize that, for the foreseeable future, I would become reac-
quainted with my feet. Here, I was always barefoot, or shod in the
plastic sandals that were the natives' basic footwear.

Yet it only took a day or two for me to understand that Carlos, Vicente, and all of the other local people around me were
going about their business in a continual state of wariness and

apprehension. Some of the threats they felt were immediate and palpable. The price of food, for example, had skyrocketed. Even rice and beans had reached luxury status. And La Libertad now operated under a curfew. Anyone in town had to be off the streets by dark. Other threats, more ominous ones, circulated as rumors. There were whispers of boys in the *mercado* being abducted by the army and forced to serve without being able to say good-bye to their families, of people disappearing in the night, even of rebels hiding in the *estero*.

My mediocre Spanish, once again rusty from lack of use, was somewhat of a barrier between me and the gruesome details. I thanked the forces of the Universe that had conspired to make me so linguistically challenged and resumed my intense practice with fervor. In the midst of constant tension, I sought stillness. Most days I found it. Hour upon hour I would meditate and practice *pranayama* and the *kriya* breath, wrapping my psyche in a cocoon of peace. I was firm in the belief that I was divinely protected and that the peace I found inside would radiate out to my environment.

On days when I had to go into La Libertad, I always asked Carlos to send word into town to send a taxi to pick me up. And it was always a relief to see the navy sentinels standing guard at the pier. I was armed with my passport, which soldiers sometimes checked. The cab waited for me as I did the shopping, and then brought me straight home. But even though my excursions were uneventful, they left me unnerved. As soon as I got back to the retreat I would work at grounding myself.

On one occasion, I came home to a tense, heated flurry of conversation between Vicente and our *guardián* as they stood listening to the radio. They snapped off the radio, and their conversation hushed when I walked by them. I never found out what they didn't want me to hear, but I knew what I needed to know: they were frightened. For a full day afterwards I, too, felt fear permeate me. No matter what I tried, I could not seem to find my center. It was a sensation that would recur from time to time when the anxiety that surrounded me was so powerful that it took on a life of its own. Even though nothing overt disturbed our world, its energy would seem to alter as the people around me, the people who comprised what had become my community, felt so obviously disengaged from the natural rhythms of their lives.

After a few months of solitude, I was joined by Walt and Magaña, who came down to check on things and to tend to paperwork entailed with the ownership of the property. I was delighted to see them, but they were gone most of each day in San Salvador, battling what had become a Kafkaesque bureaucracy. Even though Magaña was Salvadoran and still spoke Spanish fluently, it took several trips to the capital to sign some simple documents. I accompanied them on one of the trips to renew my ninety-day visa, which was about to expire. In the daylight, the third-world city seemed to have its normal chaotic atmosphere, with noisy traffic, polluted air, and masses of people going about their lives. But this surface of normalcy belied a sinister reality that was lurking in the shadows. After that trip, Gurudev warned me not to go too near the capital.

Soon after the Baptistes departed I was surprised to find I had some other visitors. The young man from the Hungry Mouth, the one who'd told me he was going to visit his uncle in the Salvadoran countryside, materialized one afternoon, with his cousin in tow. I was somewhat startled that he'd actually taken me up on my invitation and that he'd made the effort to find our isolated haven. But I invited him and his companion in with what I hoped was an air of unfettered graciousness.

My restaurant friend, Jorge, had come bearing gifts. He and

his cousin, Diego, who lived in San Salvador, had been busy digging on his uncle's land. From a clunking burlap sack they pulled a half dozen pre-Colombian artifacts. Although five of them—a little doll, a bird's head, a squirrel, and two fragments of a larger piece—had been worn by time, there was one intact bowl, a perfect relic.

"A gift for you. So you will have something of ancient El Salvador," Jorge said.

It was such a lovely gesture that I relaxed and offered the two men a glass of coco water. But as we sat and talked, I began to doubt the wisdom of my hospitality. Cousin Diego, it turned out, was a leftist guerilla who had been trained at length in Cuba. As Diego elaborated on his prowess with a variety of weapons and martial arts, it was all I could do to sit still in my chair. For the first time in years I began to think about Walt's rifle. *Where was it now? Would I need it to defend the retreat? Was this friendly visit actually a ruse for casing the property? Would our retreat become a guerilla stronghold?* I was not a political person. I didn't have enough knowledge of the complex situation to harbor sympathies one way or the other. But I did know on every level of my being that violence was the antithesis of what this sacred place was about.

Peace, harmony, well-being. Peace, harmony, well-being.

Trying to appear as casual as possible, I looked at my watch and feigned surprise at the lateness of the hour. Explaining that I had to feed the animals and water the garden and . . . and . . . whatever else I could think of, I stood up and escorted my visitors to the gate. They were perfectly polite and respectful and thanked me for the refreshments. Then, cousin Diego pulled a stubby pencil and a bit of paper from his pocket.

"Keep this number, Señorita," he said. "This is someone in the capital who can help you, if you ever need help."

I thanked them for the number and for the pottery once more and bid them good-bye. Then I watched to make sure they drove toward the highway, praying that they'd keep going.

For several weeks after the visitors came, I worried a great deal about just what I had invited into our paradise. On the face of it, I may have been guilty of nothing more than a bit of naïveté. It was doubtless not the best time to invite strangers to come and call, but when I'd encountered Jorge in the safe, faraway hubbub of the Hungry Mouth, the possible risk simply hadn't entered my mind. He was Salvadoran; I was heading to El Salvador. "Come by and see me sometime" just seemed like a natural thing to say. Still, I questioned what I'd done from a larger perspective. The cousins had roused my fear. But it was evidently lurking in the shadows, waiting to be aroused. Freud said that a fear is a wish. In a way, the karmic view is not so different: You attract from the outside what you are manifesting on the inside. Had I let fear come to the door because I was afraid to look inside and see how much of it I harbored?

The cousins never came back, but their impact lingered. I tried hard to remain alert to my own vulnerabilities. I worked at replacing fear with love, with sending love out to those around me, and to the family that I knew was so concerned for me. But some days I had the sense I'd assigned myself a Sisyphean task. I'd roll my boulder of love up the mountainside and fear would push it back down. The desperation and gloom in the air was getting to be too much for me. Still, I stayed.

One September day, after I'd been back for five months or so, I found myself alone on the beach at sunset. I had just completed several hours of deep meditation, and I calmly watched hundreds of birds cross the sky in their perfect formation. In the distance, a native fisherman appeared as a miniature figure, gazing out to sea, his trained eye keenly looking for the prize he would soon capture in his handwoven net. The sky took on a pink and lavender hue, hinting at the glorious scene that was to come as the sun slid gracefully toward the horizon. I thought to myself, *I love this place, I love this place so*. In a moment, and just for a moment, everything inside of me seemed to shift. It was as if all the love I had ever experienced in this divine setting answered me back.

I felt a rush of bliss, of gratitude, of humility. I had the rare sensation of feeling not *at* a place but truly *of* a place. I was as at home in that spot as the birds in air, and as light. But my feeling of belonging went beyond my immediate surroundings. For some reason I felt compelled to look down at my feet, and as I did so, I saw them shift their appearance as I gazed, transfixed. One instant, I was Señorita Michele in her plastic sandals; the next I was big-city Michele in her high heels. I blinked, and was barefoot once more. Who was I? I was both of these women, and I was also a woman I had barely even met yet—the one I would grow into. Where was my spiritual center? It was here on this beautiful beach, it was back in San Francisco, it was (of this I suddenly had no doubt) anywhere and everywhere I might go. My love for this haven had grown so powerful that I had been granted the great gift of carrying my home with me. I would be able always to access the oasis that was now a part of me.

And so it was settled. I called Walt the next morning and told him I was ready to go back to San Francisco, for good.

CHAPTER 21

THE CRYSTAL BALL

*"When we walk to the edge of all the light we have and take
the step into the darkness of the unknown, we must believe
that one of two things will happen. There will be something
solid for us to stand on or we will be taught to fly."*

—PATRICK OVERTON

San Francisco, June 1987

When the phone rang, an uncharacteristic ray of June sun-
light was dancing across the paperwork on my desk. I offered
my usual cheery greeting.

"Walt and Magaña Baptiste Yoga and Dance Center. Good
morning."

"Good morning to you, Michele," Walt's voice answered
back playfully. Then his tone became more serious. "I have
something important to speak with you about."

Walt was not much for small talk, and in the past six years
that I'd been working as his personal assistant, I'd gotten used
to managing Center business in an efficient way. It sounded like
Walt was calling to ask me to fill in for him at a yoga class or

to announce a change in the dance troupe schedule. I certainly didn't expect what came next.

"We're selling the building, Michele. We are currently looking for a studio to rent but we will be closing these doors in three months' time."

Wow! This was big.

"You've been doing a wonderful job here," Walt went on.

That was nice to hear.

"You do so much. You've learned so much. You are appreciated on so many levels. You are well prepared to go out into the world. And your time has come to step out into the world and teach people all that you have learned."

What?

"Gurudev," I said, "I'm not sure what you mean."

"You told me long ago you came here to become a teacher. You told me you wanted to help people find God. Raja Yoga is your path to do so. And you have something to learn about people that you must be out in the world to learn. I am giving you three months to find your next position."

I don't remember saying good-bye or hanging up, although I must have maintained my composure long enough to do so. I was utterly stunned. I had been working for Walt for thirteen years. It had not occurred to me that I would be thrown out of the nest today—or, for that matter, any day.

Since returning from El Salvador six years before and acclimating to city life once more, I had carved out an idyllic life for myself. I'd moved away from the ocean to a small jewel of a house in Marin County, high atop a ridge with a spectacular view of the bay. I'd become increasingly friendly with my neighbors on the hill, and we often enjoyed each other's company on long, lovely hikes. I had become serious in the gym, and one year I had even entered the Mr. and Ms. San Francisco Bodybuilding Competition. I was dating a man who owned a small yacht anchored at Sausalito. And at the Center, I had become Gurudev's right hand, moving with ease from managing enrollments to substituting in yoga classes, teaching at the gym, and playing flute for the dance troupe (no more waiting tables for me!). The truth was, I had been more than prepared to keep on doing exactly what I was doing indefinitely. And why not? On a subtle level, I flattered myself that I had become all but indispensable, and I saw myself there forever.

But I had forgotten one thing: a true spiritual teacher does not hold on to his students. He lets them go.

After my initial shock subsided, I began, ever so tentatively, to envision a future that did not revolve, at least in any material sense, around the Baptistes' world. I'd sit in my bay window, wide vista before me, and allow myself to scribble on a yellow legal pad anything and everything that came to mind.

"The whole world is open." I said aloud. "I can do anything, so what would I like to do?"

My resulting wish list included everything from "go to Japan" to "work on a cruise ship" to "change people's lives with yoga and meditation" to "find my soul mate." I had no idea how, or if, any of these things connected. I just put them out to the universe.

Over the next few months, I lapsed into worry every now and again, but more and more I began to feel at ease and even excited with the idea of stepping out into the world. The faith I had in the guru and his ability to see my future, even if I could not yet see it, was strong. Besides, I drew a lot of strength from what Walt had said about it being time for me to teach. A few years ago I had broached the idea of teaching a class of my own outside of the Center, and he had made it clear that, in his opinion, I was not yet up to the task. "If a yoga teacher isn't emotionally prepared and teaches out of ego," he'd said, "they can take on the karma of the entire class." That was certainly too big a bite for me to chew. It was all I could do to handle my own karma. But now that Gurudev had said I *was* ready, my confidence blossomed.

One morning, I was working in the gym with a woman named Pat, a travel agent, who had become a regular at the Center. I confided my dilemma to her.

Pat became noticeably animated as she began describing a spa in Mexico from which she had just returned. "It would be perfect for you, Michele. They have all sorts of fitness classes, several gyms, and a yoga program. You would love it there!"

It was a warm September day when I walked out of the Center for the last time. Although everyone knew I was leaving, I had declined to let them make any kind of fuss. Besides, most of the students had the daunting mission of helping move many years of accumulated treasures out of the building, a herculean task at the least. At the end of the afternoon, I quietly packed up my desk, which was filled with Walt's writings, yoga center materials, and a few cherished personal items: a mug from Norman, a crystal from Magaña.

My box of treasures did not include a crystal ball. But if it had, there is much it would have shown: a series of serendipitous events guiding me to the job teaching yoga at Rancho La Puerta, a magical fitness resort and spa in Baja California; a glorious year representing the Golden Door, the world's premier spa, on the Cunard cruise ship line—a job that took me all over the world, including Japan; opportunities to teach meditation and yoga in settings that ranged from Esalen Institute in Big Sur to universities to top medical centers; and the opportunity to work with healers like Bernard Jensen and Jonas Salk. And, at long, long last, a union with my true soul mate.

But as I say, I did not have a crystal ball. I had only my hope, my faith in God and my dear guru, and my own two feet to carry me. Armed with these things, and nothing more, I stepped out into the great unknown.

CHAPTER 22

THROUGH THE OPEN DOOR

San Francisco, August 2001

A month had passed since Gurudev's death. He died while my husband and I were planting a pear tree in our Sonoma retreat garden. "It is a part of Raja Yoga life to plant trees," he'd told us the week before.

Mehrad and I arrived at the Unitarian Church early and found a parking spot within the block—practically a miracle in itself for San Francisco. Magaña had chosen the Unitarian Church for the memorial, because she said it lent itself to the universality of all religions and philosophies, which had been one of the cornerstones of her husband's teachings. With my flute case in hand, I joined Bob and the other musicians who had set up their equipment on the right side of the altar.

I held back my tears. To cry and play my flute at the same time obviously wouldn't work. And it was more important to express my love and gratitude to Gurudev through the flute sounds that he loved so dearly than to drown in my own emotions.

I looked out into the crowded church and saw new friends and old. Many I had not seen since my days at the Center. There were some people I didn't recognize. We musicians began to play the Songs of the Teachings that were such a part of our life with Walt. Then, to the exquisite strains of the soprano's "Ave Maria," the procession of Gurudev's immediate family entered from the back of the church, led by an Episcopalian priest, a family friend, who held Walt's ashes in a small chest.

Magaña took my breath away. She was dressed in a long, simple, white caftan robe with flowing sleeves, her long, dark hair falling softly on her shoulders. When the group arrived at the altar, the priest spoke for a short time and then Magaña came to the center of the altar, carrying a Tibetan healing bowl, which she struck three times. She removed her white caftan; beneath it she wore a long black velvet dress with a simple full skirt and a long white chiffon scarf around her neck. "In sacred dance," she'd once told me, "the scarf represents another extension of the aura in a veil form. You learn to feel it with your movement as a spiritual flow, and it represents the luminescent spirit."

Then, raising the scarf to the heavens, Magaña danced for her husband and spiritual partner. She danced for each moment of their sixty years together. She danced from the depths of her soul, filling the church with her spirit and touching the souls of everyone in the room. Her movements were understated and exquisite, with spiritual sacred hand gestures that carried within them the mysteries of the universe. She danced to uplift us all.

Afterward, people close to Walt spoke. Through them a picture of a Renaissance man emerged: a practical mystic with his head in the stars and both feet planted firmly on the ground, and a great yogi who dedicated his life to teaching and serving others.

As I waited for my turn to speak, I again tried to con'
tears. My thoughts went back to the beach in El Salv
many years before, where Miguel and Maria's bodies lay empty
and Walt's words over the phone consoled me and allowed me
to fully experience my sadness. I remembered the day of the
pyramid initiation, where Walt taught us of the secret opening at
the crown of the head, the Tenth Door, and shared with us the
ancient practices for conscious dying. In my heart, I felt certain
that Walt left his body through that sacred portal and was even
at that moment on a voyage that transcended the bonds of time.

I thought, too, of the many times since leaving the Center
that Walt gave me advice when I sought it and applauded my
successes in the world.

Suddenly, it was my turn to speak. I took a deep breath and
walked to the microphone to give tribute to my beloved teacher.

"For twenty-seven years," I said, "I have had the grace and
good fortune to sit at the feet of a great master teacher. Well,
rather, I tried to sit at his feet, but he wouldn't let me. There
was too much work to be done. 'A spiritual devotee lives five
lifetimes in one,' he would often say.

"From the moment he greeted me warmly with the words
'Welcome home,' my life became unbelievably full. Along the
way Walt Baptiste guided me, he applauded me, he scolded me,
he lifted me, and he showed me how to dive into the innermost
recesses of my being.

"In the Vedas, the great yogic scriptures, there is a prayer:
'Lead me from the unreal to the real, from darkness to light,
from death to immortality.' That was what my guru did for me.
He taught me that what I perceived to be reality was so limited
compared to the deeper truth. He taught me how to traverse the
ups and downs of materiality. He taught me that I was creating

my life through the powers of my mind and the quality of my thoughts. Through him, I learned practical, down-to-earth ways to care for my body through diet and exercise so that I would have the stamina to live life to its fullest. Walt Baptiste taught me the inner secrets of yoga breathing and showed me the way to find the divine force within me. He taught me about the Laws of the Universe and how to live by them, and he taught me how to prepare for my death.

"He once said to me, 'A teacher must inspire people, Michele. Inspiration is so important!' Walt Baptiste's life inspires us all to reach beyond our common and ordinary experience—to break out of our mold, to reach for the stars. To live with passion! To think big—not just big thoughts, but great thoughts. To dream beautiful dreams and to live them out. To grow and unfold into the fullness and wholeness of all that we can be.

"Whenever I thanked Walt Baptiste for anything, he would answer, 'Thank God instead.' I thank God for Walt Baptiste."

EPILOGUE

I have no doubt that Walt Baptiste passed through the Tenth Door to embark on the ultimate journey. He had often reminded us that, to the yogi, the high purpose of meditation is to learn how to die before dying, so that at the moment of death, we will be familiar with our transition from this life as souls with bodies to our life as pure spirit. I have no way of knowing the full dimensions of that journey, except by exposing myself to the words of the great spiritual teachers who have had firsthand experience of our ultimate destination. These teachings can be found in all the great religions and wisdom traditions throughout history.

I do know one thing with certainty: my relationship to my teacher continues on uninterrupted. The relationship between the guru and student does not change after the guru transitions to the next life. During meditation, the teacher continues to guide the student on the inner planes and is continuously present in spirit for the student throughout this life and in all of the student's incarnations.

I also know for certain that within our own dimension, Walt lives on in tangible ways, through all of those whose lives he touched and who continue to pass on his teachings to others. Walt Baptiste was a Teacher of Teachers. He worked closely with his students to take them as far as they were willing to go. He encouraged us to be "practical mystics," imparting the best of our own experience in an accessible way and making the teachings applicable to the twenty-first century without diluting the essential yogic teachings and practices.

Many of the students who are a part of my story are now teaching yoga, while some are inspiring people by example in their chosen life work. An orthopedic surgeon, a musician and songwriter, a world-famous dancer, a psychologist, a playwright, a poet—all are expressing the teachings in their own unique way.

The beautiful and ageless Magaña, at eighty-nine years, continues to teach yoga classes, overflowing in capacity, in her San Francisco home, and is referred to by the press as the Grande Dame of Yoga.

The Baptiste children have all gone on to become outstanding teachers in their own right.

Baron Baptiste is one of the most sought-after yoga teachers in the U.S., has developed his own style of yoga, and teaches internationally. Devi Ananda Baptiste carries on her mother's legacy, teaching both dance and yoga in San Francisco. And Sherri Baptiste, an inspiring teacher and author, touches thousands through her Bay Area classes, teacher trainings, and international retreats.

Norman continues to serve the Baptiste legacy and is a solid presence at the Baptiste home as he registers and guides the students who arrive for Magaña's yoga classes, encouraging them onward and providing unique insights for each person's individual journey. In his eighties now, he appears to have barely aged since the day I met him in the health food store over thirty years ago.

As for me, I have never forgotten Walt's firm conviction that Raja Yoga was my path and that it was time for me to teach.

I mentioned that I finally met the soul mate I had longed for. His name is Mehrad Nazari and he has joined me on this path. One day in 1992, Walt married us in his San Francisco home, on the stairway adjacent to the large meditation room, just before the Saturday morning meditation class. During the powerful and moving ceremony, Walt rang a gigantic Tibetan bell in the four directions and placed a single garland of large *rudraksha* beads around both of our necks, joining us together.

I gazed into Gurudev's eyes and saw them brimming over with tears of love. He then gave us three pieces of wisdom regarding our marriage, which I hold close to my heart and have never forgotten. First, he advised, "Always remember that you are two separate souls and spirits." Second, "Keep each other on a pedestal." And lastly, "Practice forgiveness."

As Raja Yogis, Mehrad and I have our individual yoga practices and classes, and the central body of our work is in offering retreat experiences that we lead together. We select locations that are private, nurturing, and supportive of the spiritual intentions of the people who attend. We are both grateful to have had such personal spiritual guidance from such a great soul as Walt Baptiste, and thankful that it was our karma in this lifetime to have studied with him so closely.

Sometimes people remind me of my good fortune and lament that they have not yet met their guru or spiritual guide. Years ago, Norman told me that although some spiritual seekers may not meet their outer gurus in this lifetime, their guides are with them. Everyone has an inner guru who is waiting for them to turn inward. I wish for each of you that with an open heart, and through the practice of meditation, you will discover the teacher within who will take you by the hand and guide you through the inner door into the essence of your being: pure light, pure love, and pure joy.

SECRET CHAPTER

*T*hank you for joining for me on my spiritual adventure. If you would like a bit more, I've written a secret chapter for you that you can find at www.RajaYogis.net/secretchapter. You must log onto the page with the following password: *transform*.

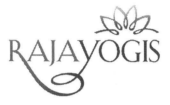

FURTHER TOOLS TO CONTINUE YOUR JOURNEY

*T*he mission of Raja Yogis (www.rajayogis.net) is to empower you to create and deepen your spiritual practice for personal transformation. We offer DVDs and CDs that bring you the practices you have read about in this book and that provide ways to expand your consciousness in meditation. For those of you interested in deepening your experience, please join us for one of our many retreats. There, among kindred spirits, you will immerse yourself in the Raja Yoga teachings and practices, gain new levels of clarity and insight, and awaken the sacred in your everyday life.

ACKNOWLEDGMENTS

My deep appreciation goes to Arlene Matthews, my collaborative editor, who organized and guided me through the complicated process of writing this book and whose gift as a wordsmith is unsurpassed. Arlene eagerly dove into the practices outlined in the book in order to have a greater understanding of Walt Baptiste's teachings.

I am eternally grateful to Walt and Magaña Baptiste for their inspiration, spiritual guidance, and unconditional love.

And to my dear mentor Norman, a truly great yogi, who continues to always be there whenever needed, and to all of the Baptiste spiritual family, with whom I share a unique life experience. I love you all for your dedication to your ideals.

To Sherri Baptiste, my spiritual sister and coworkshop leader, whose enthusiasm in passing on the teachings is boundless.

And, of course, I must thank my parents, Bill and Olive Hébert. Not only did my mother proofread the manuscript, but, hey, neither she nor my father disowned me during all those years when I was doing "Lord knows what" in El Salvador.

Mehrad Nazari, my best friend and husband, supported me throughout this project and in life in general. Mehrad found my long-lost journals in a box in the back of the garage on the very day I was beginning this book and saved me years of trying to remember.

Thank you to Deborah Szekely, the founder of Rancho La Puerta Fitness Resort, to her daughter Sara Livia Brightwood, to

Phyllis Pilgrim, and the entire Ranch family, all of whom are dedicated to creating an oasis for the spirit where I have been invited to share these teachings to many thousands of guests over a twenty-year period.

My gratitude goes to Michael Murphy, founder of Esalen Institute, and to all the Esalen family, who further the education of the human spirit and who brought me into their family of teachers.

Many thanks to Peter and Kathie Davis, founders of IDEA Health and Fitness Association and of Inner IDEA, who introduced the concept of mind, body, and spirit to the global fitness industry and gently raise the awareness of millions through their work. Peter and the following people were kind enough to read my manuscript: Dan Wakefield, Linda Johnsen, Linda Wertheimer, Meredith Brokaw, Lisa Hébert, Gay Luce, Sarah Livia Brightwood, Phyllis Pilgrim, Janice Gronvold, Rhana Pytell, Victoria Danzig, Claire Tehan, Bette Timm, Martin Hébert, Carolyn Boline, Kim Jewell, Tejas Chandaria, and, last but not least, my literary representative Winnie Kelly, who bent over backwards to get the manuscript out into the world.

Finally, a special thank you to the team at Greenleaf Book Group and to brilliant book designer Judythe Sieck, who has been encouraging me to write this book for twenty years and who lovingly designed this book's interior.

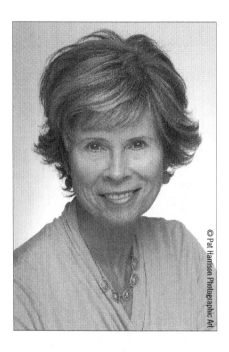

ABOUT THE AUTHOR

Michele Hébert is a leader in mind-body health and spirituality. She blends her background in yoga, fitness, meditation, nutrition, and healing to guide others in achieving higher levels of health and spiritual awareness.

As a senior teacher in the Walt Baptiste method of Raja Yoga, her work has been a transformative factor in the lives of thousands over a thirty-year period. She continues her spiritual studies with Swami Veda Bharati of Rishikesh, India, and was initiated into Tibetan Buddhism by H.H. the Dalai Lama.

Currently, Michele teaches Raja Yoga in La Jolla, California, and The Art of Meditation at the University of California, San Diego. She coleads international yoga and meditation retreats with her husband, Dr. Mehrad Nazari.

For more about Michele log onto www.rajayogis.net.

Made in the USA
San Bernardino, CA
11 June 2019